M000250538

Your Ultimate Guide to MIPS, 2018 Edition

By Joy Rios, MBA, CHTS-PW

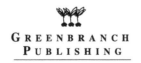

GREENBRANCH
PUBLISHING

Copyright © 2018 by Greenbranch Publishing, LLC
ISBN: 978-0-9993553-8-1
eISBN: 978-0-9993553-9-8

PO Box 208
Phoenix, MD 21131
Phone: (800) 933-3711
Fax: (410) 329-1510
Email: info@greenbranch.com
Websites: www.greenbranch.com, www.mpmnetwork.com, www.soundpractice.net

All rights reserved. No part of this book shall be reproduced, stored in a retrieval system, or transmitted by any means, i.e. electronic, mechanical, photocopying, recording, or otherwise, without written permission of the publisher. Please do not participate in or encourage piracy of copyrighted materials in violation of the authors' rights. Purchase only authorized editions. Routine photocopying or electronic distribution to others is a copyright violation. Please notify us immediately at (800) 933-3711 if you have received any unauthorized editorial from this book.

No patent liability is assumed with respect to the use of the information contained herein. Although every precaution has been taken in the preparation of this book, the publisher and the authors assume no responsibility for errors or omissions. Nor is any liability assumed from damages resulting from the use of the information contained herein. For information, Greenbranch Publishing, PO Box 208, Phoenix, MD 21131.

This book includes representations of the author's personal experiences and do not reflect actual patients or medical situations.

This book is not intended as a substitute for the medical advice of physicians. The reader should regularly consult a physician in matters relating to his/her health and particularly with respect to any symptoms that may require diagnosis or medical attention.

The strategies contained herein may not be suitable for every situation. This publication is designed to provide general medical practice management information and is sold with the understanding that neither the author nor the publisher is engaged in rendering legal, accounting, ethical, or clinical advice. If legal or other expert advice is required, the services of a competent professional person should be sought.

Greenbranch Publishing books are available at special quantity discounts for bulk purchases as premiums, fund-raising, or educational use. info@greenbranch.com or (800) 933-3711.

13   8 7 6 5 4 3 2 1

Copyedited, typeset, indexed, and printed in the United States of America

PUBLISHER
Nancy Collins

EDITORIAL ASSISTANT
Jennifer Weiss

BOOK DESIGNER
Laura Carter
Carter Publishing Studio

COPYEDITOR
Leslie Diane Poston

TABLE OF CONTENTS

ACKNOWLEDGMENTS

This book would not have been possible without support and assistance from a few key members of the Technical Director team at Inform Diagnostics. Mike Lacenere, Robin Roberts, and the entire Technical Director team have been instrumental in turning this book into a reality by examining the MIPS from both a 30,000-foot view as well from the weeds. Having such knowledgeable and experienced team members to share ideas with has been a professional dream come true.

I must also express my gratitude for the love and support of my husband and family who continue support me in my professional endeavors.

A sincere thanks to my copy editor, Leslie Diane Poston at A Draft Supreme, LLC, she's the real hero.

And to the newest member of my family who, rain or shine, makes sure I get outside, preferably to the dog park: thank you Juno.

ABOUT THE AUTHOR

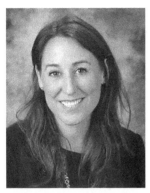

Joy Rios, MBA, CHTS-PW, is a subject matter expert and health IT consultant focusing on the Merit-based Incentive Payment System (MIPS). She has a unique talent for taking convoluted materials, such as government incentive program documentation, and distilling them down to the applicable information that healthcare professionals need to succeed.

She works as a Technical Director for Inform Diagnostics, and focuses on training a national consulting team of more than 50 professionals in an effort to support clinicians through navigating health IT initiatives. In the past, she has developed several training programs and online courses on various health IT subject areas.

Joy holds an MBA with a focus in sustainability, and is a Certified Healthcare Technology Specialist with a specialty in Workflow Redesign, as well as a Certified MACRA-MIPS Healthcare Professional. She also holds HIPAA security certification, and has been a notable resource for providers across the country navigating the new healthcare landscape. Connect with Joy online at www.twitter.com/askjoyrios or email at: joyrios@gmail.com.

EDITOR'S NOTE

The MACRA statute has two distinct tracks, both of which can take you down a proverbial rabbit hole. This book will focus on just one of those tracks: The Merit-based Incentive Payment System (MIPS). The other track is entitled the Alternate Payment Models (APMs) and the information pertaining to this track would fill a whole other book. If you're looking for in-depth guidance on APMs or even "MIPS APMs," this is not the place.

Additionally, there is no one-size-fits-all solution for clinicians for MIPS. Each organization will want to stay on top of the program to determine which routes are right for them.

While great care was taken to ensure that the information contained in this book is true and correct at the time of publication, changes in MIPS regulations and requirements will continue to be updated annually, and even semi-annually, which may impact the accuracy of this information.

INTRODUCTION

Change is hard at first, messy in the middle, and if we're lucky, gorgeous at the end. If nothing else, it certainly is an iterative process—and real change takes time.

Over the past seven years, the United States has been the site of a historic health IT transformation, transitioning from a primarily paper-based health system to one where virtually every individual has a digital footprint of their care history due to the dramatic uptick of electronic health records (EHRs). Today, nearly all hospitals (96 percent) and nearly eight in 10 (78 percent) physicians use certified EHRs. This transformation can be directly attributed to the Health Information Technology for Economic and Clinical Health (HITECH) Act of 2009; at the time it was enacted, fewer than one in 10 hospitals and just 17 percent of physicians used EHRs.

Healthcare's next major legislative push came in 2015, with the passing of the Medicare Authorization and CHIP Reimbursement Act (MACRA), which intended to jumpstart a monumental shift toward value-based care.

Information in this book will provide insight and practical strategies for a healthcare practice to navigate many of the inherent challenges that MACRA entails.

The breadth and depth of this information is complex due to the sheer size of the program, the number of clinicians subject to its requirements, and the unprecedented monetary investment in the model's approach. Add to this the fact that each participant's reputation is on the line, since all performance results will be made public, and suddenly there's pressure to act.

Think of MACRA as a mountain, with a "pick your pace" element to it. The speed at which you proceed doesn't matter as much as getting started. So let's begin the journey together, taking one step at a time.

CHAPTER 1

Welcoming a New Healthcare Paradigm

So the saying goes, when one door closes, another opens.

You may or may not know how the national healthcare system became so out of control in terms of cost and budget. It's a complex matter, but the Sustainable Growth Rate was a foundational factor. What is the Sustainable Growth Rate, you ask?

Congress established the Medicare Sustainable Grown Rate (SGR) provision as part of the Balanced Budget Act of 1997, which established a yearly monetary target for physicians' services under Medicare. Their intent was to control the cost of Medicare expenditures for services provided by physicians. The SGR target did not directly limit the services that physicians provided. Instead, each year, if the physicians' expenditures were above the target, the following year's fee schedule (i.e. how much a physician is paid for their services) would be reduced in order to compensate the difference.

Year after year, physicians' costs to the Medicare system for treating patients were consistently greater than the target. This resulted in the reimbursement rates for services decreasing for several years in a row. Think about that for a second. How would you feel if you got a pay cut after your annual review? What would you do if that happened several years in a row?

By 2015, physicians' costs were so far over the target that if Congress were to continue applying the same methodology to bring the costs back within budget, they would have had to reduce payments to physicians by 21 percent.

Instead of applying this same "doc fix," the idea of pushing healthcare away from the "fee-for-service" system and into a payment model that involves greater accountability for providers the quality and cost of the care they deliver took hold in Congress. At this point, it was clear that the Sustainable Growth Rate was not sustainable at all.

To address this issue, the Medicare Authorization and CHIP Reimbursement Act (MACRA) was introduced to Congress as a budget-neutral program, thereby eliminating the need to "fix" the model each year. In place of the SGR,

MACRA would create a systematic way to compare clinicians across the country, and pay them in accordance with their ranking.

It is worth noting that in the midst of a contentious, gridlocked Congress, on April 16, 2015 MACRA passed with bipartisan support through a vote of 392-37 in the House of Representatives and 89-7 in the Senate.

MACRA authorized the Quality Payment Program (QPP), which allows clinicians to choose how they want to participate in the program based on their practice size, specialty, location, and/or patient population under two tracks: The Merit-based Incentive Payment System (MIPS) and the Advanced Alternate Payment Models (APMs).

CMS has identified a few cornerstone elements of the new payment model that will be critical for success. These include improving patient outcomes and ensuring that all clinicians offer high quality, patient-centered care. They also feel it is important to provide meaningful feedback to clinicians so their performance can be improved where needed. CMS also believes that the program should evolve over time, leading to continuous improvement.

Additionally, CMS has issued several strategic goals as part of the QPP that build on the three cornerstones above, and include:

- Improving beneficiary outcomes
- Enhancing clinician experience
- Increasing the adoption of Advanced APMs
- Maximizing participation
- Improving data and information sharing
- Ensuring operational excellence in program implementation

Let's shine a light for a moment on the Medicare costs that have been the driver of much of this shift from a fee-for-service model toward one that pays for performance.

For context, Medicare spending represented 15 percent of the total federal budget in 2015—$632 billion—and 20 percent of total national spending in 2014.

This aligns with reality. The U.S. has an aging population, with 10,000 baby boomers enrolling in Medicare *every day*. Like all seniors, as they age, baby boomers typically increase their use of medical goods and services. This trend is expected to accelerate until around 2030, when demographers predict that all the baby boomers will have passed the age of 65.

Looking forward, net Medicare spending, defined as mandatory Medicare spending minus income from premiums and other offsetting receipts, is projected to increase from $695 billion in 2016 to $1.3 trillion in 2026, according to the Congressional Budget Office.

In addition to the increase in Medicare spending, Medicare fraud has also been an issue. While it's impossible to know how much money Medicare has lost due to fraud—estimates reach as high as $60 billion—we can look to see how much money has been recovered by CMS. In June 2016 alone, the Justice Department charged 301 people with schemes that defrauded government health programs by submitting $900 million in fraudulent health claims.

Considering the risks at stake for keeping the Medicare model as-is, it's not surprising that value-based care is on the fast track toward becoming the dominant model of care delivery and payment in the United States.

Consider these interesting statistics, according to the 2017 Progress on the Path to Value-Based Care, the second annual study commissioned by Quest Diagnostics and Inovalon (Figure 1-1).

- 94 percent of provider organizations are on a path for some form of value-based care.
- 50 percent of physician reimbursement is coming through value-based care models.

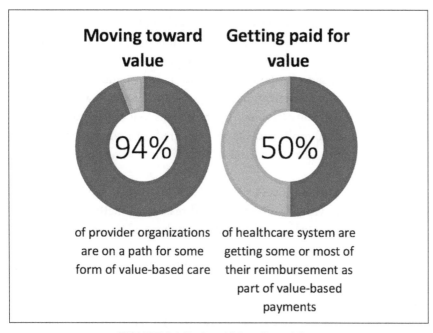

FIGURE 1-1. Path to Value-Based Care

However, challenges remain:

- 43 percent of physicians say they have the right tools to succeed under value-based care.
- 70 percent say they do not see a clear link between EHRs and better outcomes.

It is important to note that there are some links from MACRA to the Patient Protection and Affordable Care Act (ACA or "Obamacare"). However, the transition to value-based care is on track to continue regardless of changes made to the ACA by Washington.

GETTING TO KNOW MACRA

"Whether you are a patient, a provider, a business, a health plan, or a taxpayer, it is in our common interest to build a health care system that delivers better care, spends health care dollars more wisely, and results in healthier people. We believe these goals can drive transformative change, help us manage and track progress, and create accountability for measurable improvement," said Secretary Sylvia Burwell in 2015.

The U.S. Department of Health and Human Services (HHS) has set clear goals and a timeline for shifting Medicare reimbursements from volume of claims to value to patients.

This is the first time in the Medicare program's history that HHS has set explicit goals for alternative payment models and value-based payments.

The hoped for, prevailing theory is that this payment reform will ultimately drive fundamental changes in healthcare service delivery, making the entire system more responsive to those it serves and improving care coordination and communication among patients, families, and providers. MACRA and the Quality Payment Program aims to give patients and families the information, tools, and support required for them to make better-informed decisions, use their health dollars wisely, and improve health outcomes.

Until now, providers were paid for each individual service they provide—a physician visit, a surgery, a blood test, etc. Whether or not these services were over-utilized, or if they helped or harmed the patient, were not taken into account.

While I am very happy you are holding this book in your hands, I recommend you also become familiar with the Quality Payment Program website: www.qpp.cms.gov.

The QPP website allows you to review the most updated resources for the MIPS and Alternate Payment Programs, including the fact sheets for each performance category, quality measures included in the program along with their benchmarks, presentations, webinars, and a variety of other informative resources that detail different aspects of the program. The QPP website also serves as a gateway to submit MIPS data to CMS.

MACRA's budget-neutral approach introduces the concept that money collected through penalties will be redistributed to pay out incentives. It is truly a zero-sum game that rewards clinicians who play it well at the expense of clinicians who don't.

The game is played each calendar year, where all eligible clinicians will earn a score somewhere between zero and 100 points for their MIPS participation. The earned score will be used to determine their Medicare Part B reimbursement rate two years later. So, the 2017 program year will be used to determine the 2019 payment rate, the 2018 program year will be used to determine the 2020 payment rate, and so on. MACRA has been slated to take us to the 2022/2024 program and payment years.

CMS expects the majority of clinicians to participate in the MIPS track, at least for the first few years of the program. Over time, they expect that, due to the administrative burden and the financial impacts, smaller practices may close and/or providers will join larger groups that have the resources needed to be on the winning side of this game.

MAKING THE TRANSITION

In an effort to ease the transition to this new model, CMS made avoiding a penalty during the first year of participation very easy.

In 2017, clinicians had the following options:

1. Submit no data to CMS, earn 0 MIPS points, and receive an automatic 4% penalty.
2. Submit minimal data to CMS, earn 3 MIPS points, and receive a neutral payment adjustment.
3. Submit 90-days worth of data, earn up to 100 MIPS points, and receive an incentive up to 4% or more.
4. Submit data for a full calendar year, earn up to 100 MIPS points, and receive an incentive up to 4% or more.

CMS is sending a clear message: ignoring the Quality Payment program or hoping that it will just go away is an expensive attitude to adopt.

The option allowing clinicians to submit minimal data was designed to help ensure that their EHR and other systems that help collect data were working properly. It was also designed to give clinicians time to prepare for broader participation in 2018 and 2019. To avoid the penalty, those who reported MIPS in 2017 had the option to submit just one quality measure for one Medicare patient for any period of time. This "submit something" was certainly a better option than doing nothing, but it did not reflect enough effort for CMS to consider it eligible to receive an incentive in 2019.

In order to be eligible for the incentive dollars tied to 2017, a minimum of 90 days of data must have been submitted. Regarding the full calendar

MACRA's budget-neutral approach introduces the concept that money collected through penalties will be redistributed to pay out incentives. It is truly a zero-sum game that rewards clinicians who play it well at the expense of clinicians who don't.

year reporting option, CMS has recognized that physician practices of all sizes have successfully submitted a full year of quality data in past programs, and they expect that many will do so, even in MIPS' first performance year.

For the 2018 program year, CMS has extended components of the "Pick Your Pace" options in an effort to continue working toward the long-term goals of the program. The 90-day reporting option is currently only available for two of the four performance categories and this trend of the program becoming incrementally more stringent is expected to continue each year.

Since CMS expects there to be far more "losers" of this game than "winners," the incentives paid out could potentially exceed the penalties up to three times over. To put that into context, CMS predicts that for every 100 clinicians who are penalized, only about 33 will earn an incentive. With 66 "losers" contributing to a penalty fund, the *entirety* of those funds would be distributed to the 33 "winners" in the form of a higher reimbursement rate.

Then, in 2019, when each of the MIPS-eligible clinicians submit a claim for a $100 service, the 100 "losers" would receive just $96 for their service, while the 33 "winners" could receive up to $112 (Figure 1-2).

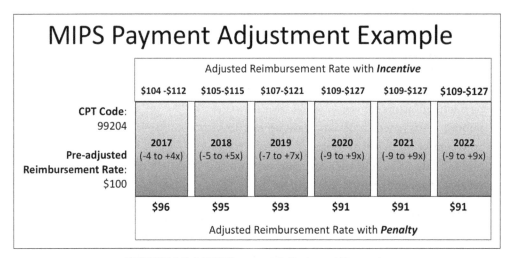

FIGURE 1-2. MIPS Payment Adjustment Example

Furthermore, Congress set aside a $500 million annual budget to be used for *additional* positive payments, on top of the budget-neutral payment adjustment, that "exceptional performers" can earn. These additional funds have the potential to be worth an additional 10 percent of your Medicare Part B billings.

Who wouldn't want to be on the winner's side of this equation? It's a triple win that yields bonus money, getting ahead of the competition, and receiving a reputation boost because, as we will detail later in this book, all of the clinicians' MIPS participation and results will be publicly available. The flip side of that coin is a triple loss, aligned with the same reasons (Figure 1-3).

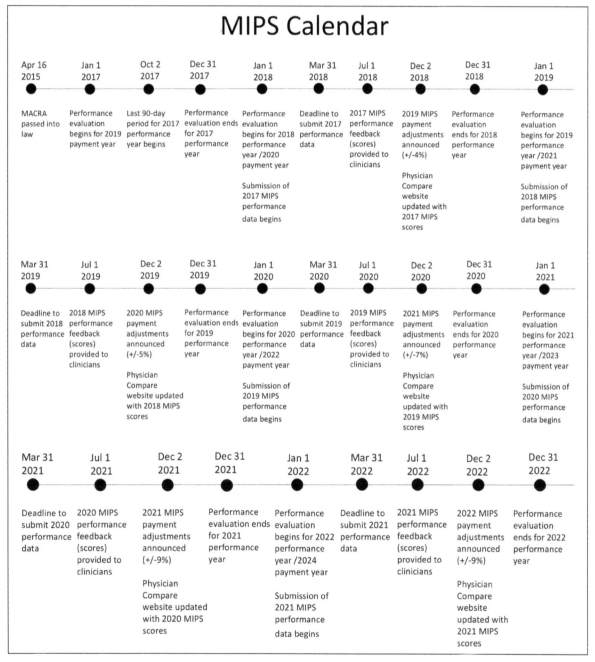

FIGURE 1-3. MIPS Calendar

Take a look at the timeline for increasing the penalties/incentives as the years pass and you'll notice that the longer the MIPS game is played, the more money is at risk. In just a few short years, the same $100 service could have a reimbursement spread of $91 to $127.

Take a look at the timeline for increasing the penalties/incentives as the years pass and you'll notice that the longer the MIPS game is played, the more money is at risk. In just a few short years, the same $100 service could have a reimbursement spread of $91 to $127.

For context, keep in mind that the above graphic only reflects Medicare reimbursements (Figure 1-4).

Also at play here is that Medicare sets the standard in the healthcare industry and among private insurance payers. Prominent insurers such as Anthem Blue Cross, United Healthcare, Aetna, and Molina to name a few, are following Medicare's lead. In fact, Anthem Blue Cross has already transitioned 60 percent of its contracts to follow the value-based model. United Healthcare has instituted a "Premium Designation" status, identifying the physicians' designation based on how they perform within the insurance company's quality and cost metrics (Figure 1-5).

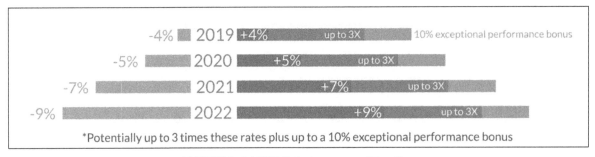

-4% ■ 2019 +4%	up to 3X	10% exceptional performance bonus
-5% 2020 +5%	up to 3X	
-7% 2021 +7%	up to 3X	
-9% 2022 +9%	up to 3X	

*Potentially up to 3 times these rates plus up to a 10% exceptional performance bonus

FIGURE 1-4. MIPS Reimbursement Timeline

Your 2018 UnitedHealth Premium Designation

Premium Specialty	Designation	Effective Date	Status	Reason	Reconsideration Due Date Prior to Effective Date
Dermatologist	Quality Care Physician	3/30/2018	Pending	Annual Assessment	1/30/2018

Please see the enclosed Overview of 2018 Premium Program for a detailed explanation of the designations for the Premium Program.

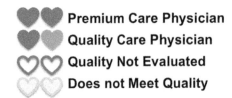

Premium Care Physician

Quality Care Physician

Quality Not Evaluated

Does not Meet Quality

Premium Program Assessment Reports
Sign in to UnitedHealthCareOnline.com to view your designation and your assessment reports.

FIGURE 1-5. Commercial Payer's Version of Value-Based Care

In the private payer world, these designations can influence an insurance company's recommendations and referrals to its patients. It can also influence the company's reimbursement rates.

What's more, value-based care is also influencing behavior at the corporate level, placing emphasis on wellness programs and preventive treatment. The thought is that an employee who does not become sick will not only gain from the health benefits, but also gain from the intrinsic benefits of lower costs throughout the healthcare system as a result of value-based care. Following in CMS's footsteps, private payers hope to reduce waste and duplication, spread clinical and operational best practices, and ultimately achieve higher quality patient outcomes for a better price.

Focusing on patient engagement and placing patients at the center of their own care is a main tenet of this value-based paradigm shift. The government has been making an effort to educate patients about their rights and responsibilities. Specifically, there is more of a push to encourage patients to access their medical records, become more informed about their health, share relevant information with people they trust (i.e. a family member or other healthcare professional), and know how to keep that information safe.

Putting these patient-based tasks through an MIPS lens, my health IT attuned eye sees a direct correlation of these activities to the Providing Patients Access, Patient Education, View, Download, Transmit (VDT), and Protecting Patient Information objectives included in the MIPS.

CHAPTER 2

MIPS Overview

The Merit-based Incentive Payment System (MIPS) combines various elements of three legacy programs into a single, improved reporting system. The last performance period for the three legacy programs was 2016. The payments that will be issued under these programs will occur in 2018.

MIPS-eligible clinicians will earn a payment adjustment based on evidence-based and practice-specific quality data (Figure 2-1). Clinicians can show they provided high quality, efficient care supported by technology by submitting information to CMS in the following categories:

- **Quality** (built from the Physician Quality Reporting System or PQRS)
- **Improvement Activities** (new category, dealing with clinical transformation)
- **Advancing Care Information** (built from the Medicare EHR Incentive Program, also known as Meaningful Use, dealing with the use of certified EHR technology)
- **Cost** (built from the Value-Based Modifier program)

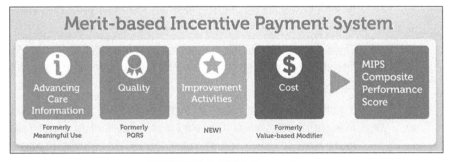

FIGURE 2-1. MIPS Categories

CMS will measure performance under these four categories and will issue a final score—somewhere between zero and 100—to each eligible clinician.

MIPS officially began on January 1, 2017 and the first performance period ran through December 31, 2017. For the first year, clinicians had the option to "Pick their Pace." This allowed them to participate as minimally or as fully as they choose. However, eligibility for an incentive payment in 2019 requires

In 2017, clinicians could avoid a penalty by earning just three MIPS points. This threshold increased to 15 MIPS points in 2018. Starting in 2019, the performance threshold will be determined annually as the mean or median of the MIPS scores for all eligible clinicians in a prior period selected by CMS. This performance threshold is expected to naturally increase year after year as average national peer performance improves and low performers potentially drop out of Medicare or MIPS entirely.

submitted data from each category for, at minimum, a 90-day period. These clinicians have until March 31, 2018 to submit their 2017 data to CMS.

Then, in July 2018, CMS will provide feedback (i.e. distribute their MIPS score) to clinicians to let them know how they performed in 2017. Beginning January 1, 2019, clinician payments from Medicare will be adjusted on a claim-by-claim basis, according to each clinician's score.

To state the obvious, a clinician's MIPS score can have a major financial impact on their practice.

In 2017, clinicians could avoid a penalty by earning just three MIPS points. This threshold increased to 15 MIPS points in 2018. Starting in 2019, the performance threshold will be determined annually as the mean or median of the MIPS scores for all eligible clinicians in a prior period selected by CMS. This performance threshold is expected to naturally increase year after year as average national peer performance improves and low performers potentially drop out of Medicare or MIPS entirely.

Another major impact of a clinician's MIPS score is reputational.

CMS will publish each eligible clinician's annual final score and the scores for each MIPS performance category within approximately 12 months after the end of the relevant performance year to the website Physician Compare (www.medicare.gov/physiciancompare).

It's mentioned that MIPS is built on the Medicare EHR Incentive Program, but there was (and still is) a Medicaid EHR incentive program that is administered voluntarily by states and territories, and will pay incentives through 2021. Eligible professionals for the Medicaid EHR Incentive Program are eligible for incentive payments for six years, where participation years do not have to be consecutive.

The last year that an eligible professional could begin participation was 2016. Incentive payments for these eligible professionals will continue to be paid out over six years.

If you qualify for both the Medicare and Medicaid EHR Incentive Programs, you must choose which program you want to participate in. If you are only eligible for the Medicaid EHR Incentive Program, you will not be subject to payment adjustments.

Medicaid eligible professionals who also treat Medicare patients will have a payment adjustment to Medicare reimbursements starting in 2015 if they do not successfully demonstrate meaningful use.

For information about the Medicaid EHR Incentive Program in previous years, visit https://www.cms.gov/Regulations-and-Guidance/Legislation/EHRIncentivePrograms/Basics.html.

Physician Compare provides useful information about physicians and other health care professionals who take part in Medicare. It exists as an effort to help consumers make informed decisions about their health and health care providers.

CMS publishes an array of clinician-identifiable performance measures through its Physician Compare website for consumers to browse and it also allows third-party physician rating websites, such as Health Grades, Yelp, and Google, to procure the published information for free. As consumers spend more out-of-pocket money for their healthcare, they are seeking more transparency in clinician quality and the cost-value equation. This site offers them a standardized way to compare clinicians in their region.

Unlike direct Medicare reimbursement impacts, which can change year to year based on clinician performance, damage to a clinician's online public reputation may take years to reverse. Conversely, consistently high performance scores and ratings could become a strategic advantage over local competitors. Think about it. If you were searching online for a doctor for your parent or for your child, would you be more likely to choose the doctor who had a rating of 3/100 or one with a rating of 80/100? Regardless of whether you understand what determines the score, if that was the only information on which to base your decision, which doctor would you select to care for your loved ones?

ELIGIBILITY

CMS determines whether a clinician needs to submit data to MIPS by looking at several criteria.

The program is so far reaching that if you have an NPI, MIPS likely applies to you.

For 2017 and 2018 (Performance Year 1 and 2), the following clinicians are included in MIPS:

- Physicians (including doctors of medicine, doctors of osteopathy, osteopathic practitioners, doctors of dental surgery, doctors of dental medicine, doctors of podiatric medicine, doctors of optometry, and chiropractors)
- Physician Assistants
- Nurse Practitioners
- Clinical nurse specialists
- Certified registered nurse anesthetists
- Groups that includes such clinicians
- (2017 only) Clinicians who billed more than $30,000 in Medicare Part B allowable charges and had more than 100 Part B-enrolled Medicare beneficiaries

> The program is so far reaching that if you have an NPI, MIPS likely applies to you.

2018 EXCLUSION CRITERIA FOR INDIVIDUAL CLINICIANS

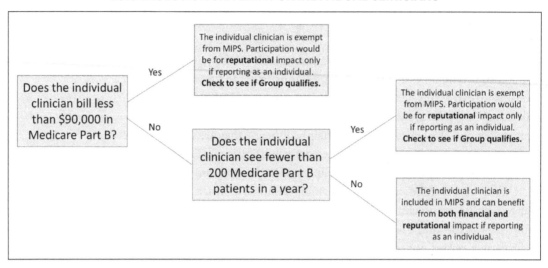

FIGURE 2-2. Exclusion Decision Tree: Individual

- (2018 only) Clinicians who billed more than $90,000 in Medicare Part B allowable charges and had more than 200 Part B-enrolled Medicare beneficiaries

In 2018, clinicians are not included in MIPS if they meet *any* of the following criteria:
- Clinicians who enroll in Medicare for the first time in 2018
- Clinicians who participate in an Advanced APM and are either a Qualifying APM Participant (QP) or Partial QP
- Clinicians who bill Medicare for $90,000 or less
- Clinicians who have provided care for 200 Medicare patients or fewer
- Clinicians who are not in a MIPS-eligible specialty

Figures 2-2 and 2-3 portray Exclusion Decision Trees: Individual and Group.

For the 2017-2018 performance years, if a clinician received 25 percent of her Medicare Part B payments through an Advanced APM or saw 20 percent of her patients, regardless of insurance payer, through an Advanced APM, she will earn a five percent incentive and MIPS exemption for the year.

During the QPP performance period, CMS will take three "snapshots" (on March 31, June 30, and August 31) to see which clinicians are participating in an Advanced APM and whether they meet the thresholds to become Qualifying APM Participants (QPs).

2018 EXCLUSION CRITERIA FOR GROUPS

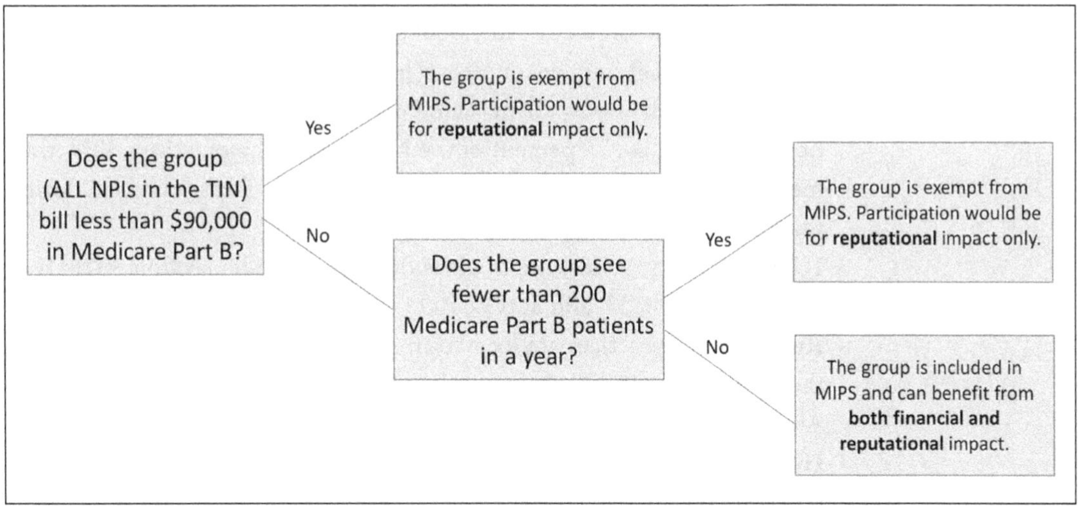

FIGURE 2-3. Exclusion Decision Tree: Group

Clinicians who participate in Advanced APMs, but don't meet the thresholds, may become Partial QPs. Partial QPs can choose if they want to participate in MIPS.

For 2017 (Performance Year 1), a clinician's eligibility was reviewed at two points in the year. If a clinician was determined exempt during the first review, she was not required to submit any MIPS data for that reporting year.

CMS completed the first review in December 2016 by examining claims from September 1, 2015 through August 31, 2016. They reviewed Medicare Part B Claims data and PECOS data, and applied their findings to 2017 (Performance Year 1).

CMS completed the second review in December 2017 by examining Medicare Part B Claims data from September 1, 2016 through August 31, 2017 and PECOS data. If a clinician joined a new practice during this time period, her eligibility under that practice was evaluated during the second review.

To check a clinician's MIPS participation status, go to the QPP website and enter your 10-digit National Provider Identifier (NPI) number. https://qpp.cms.gov/participation-lookup.

CMS offers "Special Status" to some clinicians, which means special rules under the QPP affect the number of total measures, activities, or entire categories that an individual clinician or group with "Special Status" must report. These circumstances are applicable for clinicians in: Health Professional Shortage Area (HPSA), Rural, Non-patient facing, Hospital based, and Small Practices, defined as:

- **Small Practice:** The practice that the clinician is billing under has 15 or fewer clinicians.
- **Non-patient facing:** The individual clinician has 100 or fewer Medicare Part B patient-facing encounters (including Medicare telehealth services) during the non-patient facing determination period OR the practice has more than 75 percent of the NPIs under the practice's TIN, thus meeting the definition of an individual non-patient facing clinician during the non-patient facing determination period.
- **HPSA:** These practices are in areas designated under section 332(a)(1)(A) of the Public Health Service Act.
- **Rural:** These practices are located in zip codes designated as rural, using the most recent Health Resources and Services Administration (HRSA) Area Health Resource File data.
- **Hospital-based:** The individual clinician furnishes 75 percent or more of his covered professional services in the inpatient hospital, on-campus outpatient hospital, or emergency room settings (based on place of service codes) during the applicable determination period OR all clinicians associated with the practice are hospital-based, provided that 75 percent or more of the practice's covered professional services are furnished in the inpatient hospital, on-campus outpatient hospital, or emergency room settings (based on place of service codes) during the applicable determination period.

For non-patient facing MIPS-eligible clinicians, these calculations are run twice using the same timeframe for claims of service that is used to determine whether clinicians fall below the low volume thresholds.

- September 1—August 31 of the year prior to the performance year
- September 1—August 31 overlapping the start of the performance year

If the two calculations to determine any of these special, non-patient facing status circumstances differ from one from another, the clinician or practice will receive the special status. So, for example, if a clinician met the threshold in the first timeframe, but not the second (or vice versa), she would still receive the special status from CMS.

In some instances, clinicians and groups can qualify for a hardship exemption from the MIPS categories that require the use of Certified Electronic Health Record Technology (CEHRT). This would result in reweighting the Advancing Care Information category score to zero percent of the final score if they meet the criteria outlined below. The 25 percent weighting of the Advancing Care Information category would be reallocated to the Quality category.

However, simply lacking CEHRT does not qualify the MIPS-eligible clinician or group for reweighting.

An MIPS-eligible clinician or group may submit a Quality Payment Program Hardship Exception Application, citing one of the following specified reasons for review and approval:

- Insufficient Internet Connectivity
- Extreme and Uncontrollable Circumstances
- Lack of Control over the availability of CEHRT

The deadline to submit the hardship application is December 31 of each program year.

REPORTING OPTIONS

The MACRA statute allows clinicians to choose whether they will participate in MIPS as an individual, a group, a virtual group, or under an APM entity.

Each clinician and practice must carefully evaluate how best to complete the requirements for MIPS.

Eligible clinicians must understand that the TIN/NPI combination will serve as their unique payment adjustment ID. This combination can uniquely identify every clinician, regardless of how they choose to participate, which is vital to ensure the clear accountability and portability of each MIPS score.

Individual Clinician Reporting:

If you report as an individual, your payment adjustment will be based on your performance.

An individual is defined as a single clinician, identified by a single National Provider Identifier (NPI) number tied to a single Tax Identification Number (TIN).

You'll need to send your individual data for each MIPS category through an EHR or registry. You can also send in Quality data through your routine Medicare claims process.

For 2018, you'll be able to pick from a selection of ways to submit, including:

- Qualified Clinical Data Registry (QCDR)
- Registry
- EHR
- Administrative claims
- Attestation

A group's performance is scored collectively and each physician participating in the group will earn the same MIPS final score—and the same payment adjustment.

Groups of clinicians practicing under the same TIN may report individually if all clinicians in the TIN report as individuals.

Group Reporting:

Under MIPS, a group is defined by a single TIN with two or more eligible clinicians (including at least one MIPS-eligible clinician), as identified by their NPI, who have reassigned their medical billing rights to the TIN.

Group reporting essentially treats all clinicians (MIPS-eligible and non-eligible) in the group as if they were one individual. All eligible patient encounters for each clinician in the group are aggregated together as a total population for the Quality and ACI categories (i.e. measure denominators), and each clinician's performance in the group is aggregated (i.e. measure numerators) (Figure 2-4).

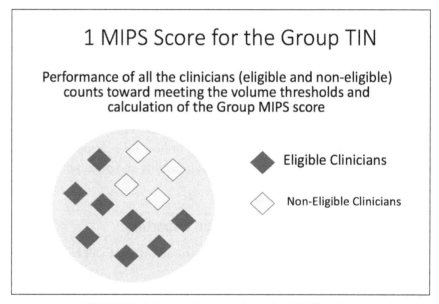

1 MIPS Score for the Group TIN

Performance of all the clinicians (eligible and non-eligible) counts toward meeting the volume thresholds and calculation of the Group MIPS score

◆ Eligible Clinicians

◇ Non-Eligible Clinicians

FIGURE 2-4. Group Reporting Includes All Clinicians

For the Quality category, the group must select six total measures to report, one of which must be an outcome measure.

For the ACI category, the group works together to meet the Base measure requirements, and can choose which measures in the Performance score to complete.

For the Improvement Activities category, the group is required to attest once the activity or activities are completed.

A group's performance is scored collectively and each physician participating in the group will earn the same MIPS final score—and the same payment adjustment.

Clinicians practicing under more than one TIN: If a clinician of a group also bills under multiple TINs, she is responsible for meeting the MIPS requirements under *each* TIN. Only services billed under a particular TIN that is reporting as a group will be included in the group's MIPS score. Services billed under different TINs may be reported individually or as a group (with the other TIN).

Reporting as a group does not affect or change the way the MIPS Composite Performance Score is calculated. The main difference is that your entire group will have their scores averaged for each MIPS category. The average score will be the group's score and will be compared against the MIPS threshold to determine the group's payment adjustment.

For 2018, groups are able to pick from a selection of ways to submit, including:
- CMS Web Interface (available to groups of 25+ eligible clinicians)
- QCDR
- Registry
- EHR
- Administrative claims
- CAHPS for MIPS Survey (available to groups of 2+ eligible clinicians)
- Attestation

There is currently no formal process for registering as a group with CMS, unless you plan to use the CMS Web Interface or report CAHPS for MIPS. Groups who want to participate in the CMS Web Interface or CAHPS for MIPS can register to do so with CMS between April 1 and June 30, 2018.

If you choose to report as a group, all clinicians billing under the TIN must report as part of the group for every MIPS category. However, certain exclusions apply to clinicians who are not MIPS-eligible. They include:
- Advanced APM participants: If a clinician billing under a TIN that elects group reporting participates in an Advanced APM, her performance is excluded from the group and the group payment adjustments will not impact the APM participant.
- New Medicare providers: Clinicians in their first year of billing Medicare are excluded from group reporting and payment adjustments.

If a clinician within the group meets the low-volume threshold exemption under MIPS (i.e. bills less than $90,000 or sees fewer than 200 Medicare patients in a year), and if together, the group exceeds the threshold, she will be included in the group and receive the same score and payment adjustment as all other clinicians in the group.

Virtual Group Reporting

Virtual groups are a relatively new concept, so let's take a closer look.

A virtual group is a combination of two or more TINs made up of one or more solo practitioners or one or more groups consisting of 10 or more clinicians (including at least one MIPS-eligible clinician), or both, that elect to form a virtual group for a one-year performance period.

To be eligible to join a virtual group, you must be a:

- **solo practitioner** who exceeds the low-volume threshold; and who is not a newly Medicare-enrolled eligible clinician, a Qualifying APM Participant (QP), or a Partial QP choosing not to participate in MIPS.
- **group** that exceeds the low-volume threshold at the group level (i.e. the NPIs within the TIN collectively exceed the low-volume threshold) and has 10 or fewer clinicians (including at least one MIPS-eligible clinician).

You can participate in a virtual group if you're a:

- **clinician** type eligible for MIPS.
- **solo practitioner** who exceeds the low-volume threshold; and who is not a newly Medicare-enrolled eligible clinician, a Qualifying APM Participant (QP), or a Partial QP not choosing to participate in MIPS.
- **group** that exceeds the low-volume threshold at the group level (i.e. the NPIs within the TIN collectively exceed the low-volume threshold).

A solo practitioner or group can only participate in one virtual group in any performance period. But there are no limits on how many solo practitioners and groups can join a virtual group.

If a group chooses to join a virtual group, all of the eligible clinicians in that group must be included in the virtual group. Any group that wants to be part of a virtual group must have 10 or fewer eligible clinicians.

A whole TIN participates in a virtual group, including each clinician with an NPI under the TIN. The entire TIN will be assessed and scored together as part of the virtual group, but only the clinicians in the TIN who are eligible for MIPS can receive a MIPS payment adjustment. TIN sizes are based on how many NPIs bill under a TIN, including the clinicians who don't meet the definition of a MIPS-eligible clinician as individuals and can't participate in MIPS.

Forming a virtual group involves a two-stage virtual group election process:

- **Stage 1 (optional):** If you're a solo practitioner or a group with 10 or fewer eligible clinicians, you can choose to contact your Quality Payment Program Technical Assistance representative. Your representative can help you figure out if you're eligible to join or form a virtual group before you:

1. Make any formal written agreements.
2. Send in your formal election registration.
3. Budget your resources for your virtual group.

For groups that don't participate in Stage 1 of the election process and don't ask for an eligibility determination, CMS will see if they're eligible to be in a virtual group during Stage 2 of the election process.

- **Stage 2 (required):** As part of the Stage 2 election process, a virtual group must have a formal written agreement between each solo practitioner and group that composes the virtual group prior to submitting an election to CMS. Each virtual group must name an official representative who is responsible for submitting the virtual group's election via e-mail to MIPS_VirtualGroups@cms.hhs.gov by December 31, prior to the performance period the virtual group would like to be evaluated for in this manner.

If all criteria for forming a virtual group are met, CMS will contact the virtual group's representative and provide the virtual group with a performance identifier. **Table 2-1 details the pros and cons of reporting as a virtual group.**

Each clinician and practice must carefully evaluate how best to complete the requirements for MIPS. The MIPS program is customizable, with many options for measures, submission methods, and flexible reporting periods for the ACI and IA categories in the 2018 performance year. These factors will impact each practice differently.

There is no one-size-fits-all formula to determine who should report as a group and who should report individually.

Here are a few ideas to help you make your decision:

- Determine your goals for the 2018 performance period. Are you reaching for a bonus in 2020 or just looking to avoid the penalty? If you simply want to submit a minimum amount of data and avoid the penalty, it may not be worth changing administrative processes, so it may be easier to submit some data individually. If you are aiming for full participation and a bonus, group reporting may reduce the administrative burden and make meeting the requirements easier.
- Review the performance of every Medicare provider in your group and determine each participant's strengths and weaknesses in the previous programs (PQRS and Meaningful Use).
- Identify the submission method you plan on using for MIPS. If you do not have an EHR and plan to report Quality data through claims, the group reporting option is not available to you. Make sure you have the requisite systems in place to participate as a group.

TABLE 2-1. Pros and Cons of Reporting as a Virtual Group

Pros	Cons
There is shared responsibility and risk.	Electing to report as a virtual group is irrevocable for one performance period.
Shared resources can support and positively impact performance in the MIPS.	It is difficult to aggregate data across disparate systems for unified reporting of MIPS measures and activities
Virtual groups would allow clinicians and groups from different TINs to participate, even if they don't meet the MIPS participation threshold individually.	Control of the virtual group's success will be in the hands of an administrator who may not be part of your practice.
There is collective potential to improve care coordination, and subsequently improve health outcomes.	There are logistical challenges in trying to manage groups that are working in different systems, geography, and reporting structures.
	Your practice will suffer if another virtual group member does not optimize their participation, bringing down the overall virtual group's score that is then assigned to every member of the virtual group.
	Combining groups that are patient-facing with others that are hospital-based and/or non-patient facing could impact the ACI category, either positively or negatively. Ultimately, it means that each member has even less control over this portion of the MIPS score that will affect future payments.
	Consider existing contractual obligations with other provider organizations and groups that might impact forming a virtual group.
	Clinicians may be unaware of their obligation to participate in the virtual group, especially if it has to support many TINs. The addition or departure of eligible clinicians within a TIN could prove difficult to manage relative to their obligation to participate in the virtual group, which could affect the TIN's eligibility to continue in the virtual group in subsequent performance years.
	Audits could be a logistical nightmare.

- Group reporting is likely a good idea for clinicians who all score very similarly in the MIPS categories. In this case, the average score amongst all the clinicians would be pretty much the same as it would have been had they reported individually. The advantage would be less administrative time and paperwork. The person assigned to submitting the group's data would only need to submit once on behalf of all clinicians. It would also be easier to predict the payment adjustments across the practice, since everyone would receive the same payment adjustment percentage.

- Group reporting may also be a good idea if you have some heavy hitters in your group who bring in a lot of Medicare Part B dollars, but who are struggling under MIPS. Let's assume your practice is set up where each clinician is paid out of a pool of shared money. If you have one clinician (Dr. A) who bills $1M per year (but scores poorly in the MIPS categories), and another clinician (Dr. B) who bills $100K per year (but scores extremely well in the MIPS categories), it may be advantageous to average the group's score so that Dr. A receives a better MIPS composite performance score.

- On the other hand, if you have a lot of heavy hitters who score well under MIPS, and others who do not (such as mid-levels), reporting as a group may not be so advantageous. Instead, each clinician may want to report individually.

- Also, consider that your group payment adjustment will apply to the entire group, including new clinicians who were not in your group during the performance year. If you are thinking of growing your practice and you received a payment adjustment as a group, that may be a big deterrent.

Regardless of how you chose to report, your MIPS score will always be linked to your NPI. Even if you change groups, form a new group, or choose to report as an individual instead of part of a group, your MIPS score will remain with you. You *will* receive the positive or negative payment adjustment based on your performance year MIPS score.

If you happen to have multiple MIPS scores (under different entities) for a single performance year, the payment adjustment will be based on the highest MIPS scores you earn.

CHANGES TO SCORING BY YEAR

Providers would be wise to take the 2017 and 2018 program years to better understand the Cost category in order to proactively and positively impact their MIPS score in future years, as this category will eventually make up 30 percent of the score (Figure 2-5).

CMS will specify a performance threshold for each MIPS payment year. For the 2017 program year, clinicians could avoid a negative payment adjustment if they received a MIPS score of three or above. For the 2018 program year, the threshold to avoid a negative payment adjustment has increased to 15.

Earn 15 points = Avoid Penalty

Earn 15 points = Avoid Penalty

Earn 70+ MIPS points = Exceptional Performance

A final MIPS score of 100 can earn an *additional* 10 percent adjustment to Medicare Part B reimbursements.

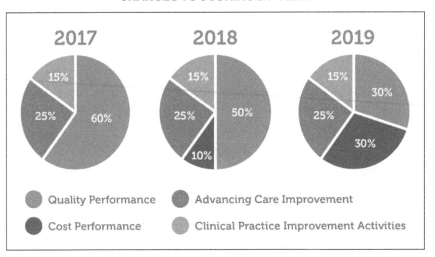

CHANGES TO SCORING BY YEAR

FIGURE 2-5. MIPS Category Scores by Year

In the 2019 program year and beyond, CMS will use either the mean or the median final score from a prior MIPS reporting period as the threshold.

In addition to the traditional upward payment adjustment that mirrors the downward one, CMS has built in an additional performance threshold where clinicians can earn even more incentive money for achieving a score above 70 points (for both the 2017 and 2018 program years), which CMS considers "exceptional performance." The reward for achieving an exceptional score is an additional adjustment factor starting at 0.5 percent and increasing, on a linear sliding scale, up to 10 percent for a final score of 100.

In the 2017 and 2018 program years, the additional performance threshold is 70 points.

Earn 70+ MIPS points = Exceptional Performance

A final MIPS score of 100 can earn an *additional* 10 percent adjustment to Medicare Part B reimbursements.

MIPS APMS

Some clinicians will find that they participate in certain types of Alternate Payment Models (APM), but also qualify for MIPS, because they did not meet the payment or patient thresholds required for exclusion from the MIPS track altogether. These clinicians are called MIPS APMs.

CMS has made an effort to ensure that the eligible clinicians in APM Entity groups are not assessed in multiple ways on the same performance activities.

If you're in a specific type of APM called a "MIPS APM" and you are not excluded from MIPS, you may be scored using a special APM scoring standard. The APM scoring standard is designed to account for activities that are already required by the APM. For example, in most cases, the APM scoring standard eliminates the need for MIPS clinicians to duplicate submission of both the Quality and Improvement Activity performance category data and allows them to focus instead on the goals of the APM.

MIPS APMs meet the following criteria:

1. APM Entities participate in the APM under an agreement with CMS or by law or regulation.
2. APM Entities include at least one MIPS-eligible clinician on a Participation List.
3. The APM bases payment incentives on performance (either at the APM Entity or eligible clinician level) on cost/utilization and quality measures.

For the 2018 performance year, clinicians who participate in any of the following models are considered MIPS APMs:

- Medicare Shared Savings Program Tracks 1, 2, and 3
- Comprehensive ESRD Care (CEC) Model (Two-Sided Risk)
- Comprehensive Primary Care Plus (CPC+) Model
- Next Generation ACO Model
- Oncology Care Model (OCM)
- Comprehensive Care for Joint Replacement (CJR) Payment Model (Track 1-CEHRT)

The following APM scoring standard is applied to MIPS APMs (Table 2-2–2.4).

TABLE 2-2. Medicare Shared Savings Program (All Tracks) under the APM Scoring Standard

Performance Category	Reporting Requirement	Performance Score	Weight
Quality	ACOs submit quality measures to the CMS Web interface on behalf of their participating MIPS-eligible clinicians.	The MIPS quality performance category requirements and benchmarks will be used to score quality at the ACO level.	50%
Cost	MIPS clinicians will not be assessed on cost.	N/A	0%
Improvement Activities	No additional reporting necessary.	CMS will assign the same IA score to each APM Entity group based on the activities required of participants in the Shared Savings Program.	20%
Advancing Care Information	All ACO participant TINs in the ACO submit under this category according to the MIPS group reporting requirements.	All of the ACO participant TIN scores will be aggregated as a weighted average based on the number of MIPS clinicians in each TIN to yield one APM entity group score.	30%

TABLE 2-3. Next Generation ACO Model under the APM Scoring Standard

Performance Category	Reporting Requirement	Performance Score	Weight
Quality	ACOs submit quality measures to the CMS Web interface on behalf of their participating MIPS-eligible clinicians.	The MIPS quality performance category requirements and benchmarks will be used to score quality at the ACO level.	50%
Cost	MIPS clinicians will not be assessed on cost.	N/A	0%
Improvement Activities	No additional reporting necessary.	CMS will assign the same IA score to each APM Entity group based on the activities required of participants in the Next Generation ACO Model.	20%
Advancing Care Information	Each MIPS clinician in the APM Entity group reports advancing care information to MIPS through either group reporting at the TIN level or individual reporting.	CMS will attribute one score to each MIPS clinician in the APM Entity group. This score will be the highest score attributable to the TIN/NPI combination of each MIPS-eligible clinician, which may be derived from either group or individual reporting. The scores attributed to each MIPS-eligible clinician will be averaged to yield a single APM Entity group score.	30%

TABLE 2-4. All Other MIPS APMs under the APM Scoring Standard

Performance Category	Reporting Requirement	Performance Score	Weight
Quality	The APM Entity group will not be assessed on quality under MIPS in the first performance period.	N/A	0%
Cost	MIPS clinicians will not be assessed on cost.	N/A	0%
Improvement Activities	No additional reporting necessary.	CMS will assign the same IA score to each APM Entity group based on the activities required of participants in the MIPS APM.	25%
Advancing Care Information	Each MIPS clinician in the APM Entity group reports advancing care information to MIPS through either group reporting at the TIN level or individual reporting.	CMS will attribute one score to each MIPS clinician in the APM Entity group. This score will be the highest score attributable to the TIN/NPI combination of each MIPS-eligible clinician, which may be derived from either group or individual reporting. The scores attributed to each MIPS-eligible clinician will be averaged to yield a single APM Entity group score.	75%

If you participate in two or more MIPS APMs, CMS will use the highest final score to calculate your MIPS payment adjustment with the exception of those MIPS clinicians who participate in the Medicare Shared Savings Program and the Comprehensive Primary Care Plus (CPC+) model. In these instances, you will follow the Medicare Shared Savings Program MIPS APM reporting and scoring requirements under the APM scoring standard and will not receive the CPC+ APM entity score. Instead, you will receive the Medicare Shared Savings Program ACO or participant TIN score.

Clinicians who are eligible for multiple APMs cannot receive incentives through each one. They can earn through one APM or the other, but not both.

If you participate in an APM, ensure your eligibility and understand the requirements and obligations of your specific program.

> Clinicians who are eligible for multiple APMs cannot receive incentives through each one. They can earn through one APM or the other, but not both.

Lessons Learned from the Field

Lesson 1: Pay Attention to "Snapshots"!

A practice participating in the Oncology Care Model (OCM) hired two new doctors to the practice in the 2017 program year. The first was hired in late August, the second in early September.

To be counted as a Qualifying Participant in the OCM, the clinicians needed to be associated with the practice during CMS's look-back "snapshot" by August 31, 2017.

The first new doctor made the cutoff and was categorized as a MIPS APM, along with the rest of the established clinicians in the practice. The second new doctor did *not* make the cutoff and had to submit as a traditional MIPS-eligible clinician.

The practice administrator was not aware of this factor until October, which resulted in more of an administrative burden on the staff in their efforts to collect the necessary data.

Lesson 2: If you participate in an APM, ensure the eligibility of each clinician and understand the requirements and obligations of your specific program.

A three-doctor dermatology practice signed up with a NextGen ACO at the end of 2016 so that its clinicians would be included in the APM track for the 2017 program year. However, they hired a new doctor toward the end of the 2016 calendar year and another one in the summer of 2017 and did not notify the ACO. By the time they realized that these two clinicians were not included in the ACO, but were instead eligible to report MIPS, it put their entire staff in "fire drill" mode to ensure that they collected enough data to report a 90-day period.

CHAPTER 3

Getting to 100

MIPS started for all eligible clinicians on January 1, 2017 and is comprised of four main categories that, together, will comprise your total MIPS score—somewhere between zero and 100 points. Each category has a maximum number of points that can contribute to the total score.

Let's break them down.

Quality: It's adapted from and improved upon the Physician Quality Reporting System (PQRS). This category requires clinicians to report six quality measures to CMS. There are nearly 300 measures to choose from with 80 percent tailored to specialists.

Advancing Care Information (ACI): It is built upon and adapted from the Medicare EHR Incentive Program, also known as Meaningful Use. This category measures a clinician's use of her certified EHR. At minimum, clinicians must report on four (or five) objectives (depending on their EHR version) to show that technology is implemented and being used effectively in the practice.

Cost: This category is adopted from the Value-based Modifier Program and has a reporting requirement. It assesses clinician cost performance based on Medicare claims data.

IA: This is a new performance category for clinicians. IA measures performance by assessing improvement activities focused on care coordination, beneficiary engagement, and patient safety, among others.

Your efforts in each of these categories will be combined into a single submission and reported to the government each year, to earn a MIPS Composite Performance Score.

Each performance category is scored separately as a percentage of maximum possible performance within that category. The category-level scores are then weighted as detailed in the bulleted list here (for 2017) and then summed to produce the MIPS final score.

With a nod to flexibility and multiple paths to success, CMS is offering several reporting options to achieve a final MIPS score of 100.

For the majority of eligible clinicians in the 2017 and 2018 performance years, the maximum number of points that can be earned in each MIPS category is outlined below. For the first years of the program, Quality comprises the bulk of the score, up to 60 points in 2017 and 50 points in 2018. As you can see, the Cost category did not contribute to the score in 2017, but will be worth up to 10 points in 2018. The Advancing Care Information category can earn up to 25 points and the Improvement Activities category can earn up to 15 points.

Here is where you get to choose your own adventure. Since the majority of the MIPS score is earned from the Quality category, let's begin there.

QUALITY

The Quality category feels new, but the reporting aspect has actually been used by CMS for more than a decade. As mentioned, it is based on the foundations laid by the Physician Quality Reporting System (PQRS) that was in place from 2006 through 2016. The PQRS was a reporting program intended to track certain aspects of the quality of care of Medicare patients. In the program, providers were incentivized to report their results of any *nine* approved quality measures, covering at least three National Quality Strategy (NQS) domains for 50 percent of their eligible Medicare patients (Figure 3-1).

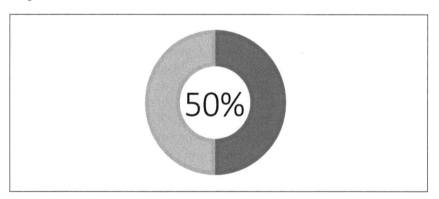

FIGURE 3-1. 2018 Quality Weight

Now, the Quality category of MIPS takes a similar approach. Generally speaking, eligible clinicians are incentivized to report the results of any *six* approved quality measures. CMS no longer requires a certain count of NQS domains be covered, although the domains still exist and come into play in other ways. And for most reporting scenarios, CMS expanded the "data completeness" requirements to include ALL relevant patients in their reporting, whether the patient uses Medicare or other private insurance payers.

Once all eligible clinicians submit their measures, CMS uses a systematic approach to benchmark their performance, or in other words, to assign a score.

To help build a more complete picture, let's take a moment to review some background information on quality measures.

Where Measures Come From

Quality measures create an objective assessment of how well healthcare providers adhere to evidence-based standards of care to achieve desired outcomes. Developed by medical professionals, the majority of quality measures originate from the American Medical Association's Physician Consortium for Performance Improvement (AMA PCPI) and are vetted by the National Quality Forum (NQF). As required by federal law, each year's list of approved measures is developed through formal notice-and-comment rulemaking. To be accepted to the list, each proposed quality measure must meet the following criteria:

- Have been adopted or endorsed by a consensus organization, such as the NQF or the Ambulatory Quality Association (AQA)
- Include measures that have been submitted by a physician specialty
- Be identified by CMS as having used a consensus-based process for development
- Include structural measures, such as the use of EHRs and electronic prescribing technology

Once accepted to the list, measures are classified against six domains, based on the National Quality Strategy's six priorities, as follows:

(1) **Patient Safety**. These are measures that reflect the safe delivery of clinical services in all healthcare settings. These measures may address a structure or process that is designed to reduce risk in the delivery of healthcare or measure the occurrence of an untoward outcome, such as adverse events and complications of procedures or other interventions.

(2) **Person and Caregiver-Centered Experience and Outcomes**. These measures reflect the potential to improve patient-centered care and the quality of care delivered to patients. They emphasize the importance of collecting patient-reported data and the ability to impact care at the individual patient level, as well as the population level. These measures of organizational structures or processes that foster both the inclusion of persons and family members as active members of the health care team and collaborative partnerships with providers and provider

organizations, can be measures of patient-reported experiences and outcomes that reflect greater involvement of patients and families in decision making, self-care, activation, and understanding of their health conditions and their effective management.

(3) **Communication and Care Coordination**. These are measures that demonstrate appropriate and timely sharing of information and coordination of clinical and preventive services among health professionals in the care team and with patients, caregivers, and families to improve appropriate and timely patient and care team communication. They may also be measures that reflect outcomes of successful coordination of care.

(4) **Effective Clinical Care**. These measures reflect clinical care processes closely linked to outcomes based on evidence and practice guidelines or measures of patient-centered outcomes of disease states.

(5) **Community/Population Health**. These are measures that reflect the use of clinical and preventive services and achieve improvements in the health of the population served. They may be measures of processes focused on primary prevention of disease or general screening for early detection of disease that are unrelated to current or prior condition.

(6) **Efficiency and Cost Reduction**. These measures reflect efforts to lower costs and to significantly improve outcomes and reduce errors. These are measures of cost, resource use, and appropriate use of healthcare resources or inefficiencies in healthcare delivery.

Defining Quality Measures

When a clinician selects a quality measure to report, the submission is expressed as a performance rate, made up of both a numerator and a denominator.

Numerator: the upper portion of a fraction used to calculate a rate, proportion, or ratio. The numerator must detail the specific clinical action required by the measure for performance. Eligible Professionals (EPs) may use the codes present in the numerator to report the outcome of the action as indicated by the measure. Quality measure numerators can be indicated with Quality Data Codes (QDCs) consisting of specified non-payable CPT Category II codes and/or temporary G-codes. For registry and electronic reporting using an EHR, other clinical coding sets may be included such as Systematized Nomenclature of Human Medicine (SNOMED), Logical Observation of Identifiers, Names, and

Codes (LOINC), or RxNorm, to capture a specific quality action, test, or value.

Denominator: the lower portion of a fraction used to calculate a rate, proportion, or ratio. The denominator must describe the population eligible (or episodes of care) to be evaluated by the measure. This should indicate age, condition, setting, and timeframe (when applicable). Quality measure denominators are identified by International Classification of Diseases, 9th Revision (ICD-9-CM) (the future ICD-10-CM), CPT Category I, and Healthcare Common Procedure Coding System (HCPCS) codes, as well as patient demographics (age, gender, etc.), and place of service (if applicable). For registry and electronic reporting using an EHR, other clinical coding sets may be included such as SNOMED, LOINC, or RxNorm.

Most quality measures are expressed in performance rates, with the numerator indicating how many times the measure has been met and the denominator indicating the opportunities to meet the measure.

For example, let's say your practice wants to measure how well it is complying with annual comprehensive foot exam recommendations for its diabetic patients. In this example, the annual foot exam would be the numerator and the number of diabetic patients seen within the year would be the denominator. The clinician's performance rate for this measure would entail calculating how many of the diabetic patients seen in the calendar year had their annual foot exam (Figure 3-2).

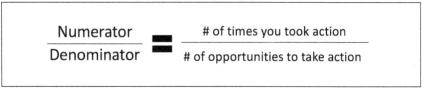

FIGURE 3-2.

Calculating Quality Measures

Calculating the quality measure's reporting rate consists of dividing the number of reported numerator outcomes by denominator-eligible encounters. The reporting rate identifies the percentage of a defined patient population that was reported for a measure. For performance rate calculations, some patients may be subtracted (i.e. excluded) from the denominator based on medical, patient, or system performance exclusions allowed by the measure.

The final performance rate calculation represents the eligible population that received a particular process of care or achieved a particular outcome. It is important to review and understand each measure's specification, as it contains definitions and specific instructions for reporting the measure.

Determining a Quality Measure's Reporting Frequency

Each measure specification sheet includes a reporting frequency for each denominator-eligible patient seen during the reporting period. The reporting frequency described in the measure specification's instructions applies to both individual clinicians and those reporting as a group. The reporting frequency is used in analyzing each measure to help determine satisfactory reporting according to the reporting frequency in the "instructions" section of the measure. The following types of reporting frequencies can be included in a quality measure's specification sheet:

- *Patient-Process*: Report a minimum of once per reporting period per individual eligible clinician.
- *Patient-Intermediate:* Report a minimum of once per reporting period per individual eligible clinician. The most recent quality action is utilized for performance calculations.
- *Patient-Periodic:* Report once per timeframe specified in the measure for each individual eligible clinician during the reporting period.
- *Episode:* Report once for each occurrence of a particular illness/condition by each individual eligible clinician during the reporting period.
- *Procedure:* Report each time a procedure is performed by the individual eligible clinician during the reporting period.
- *Visit:* Report each time the patient is seen by the individual eligible clinician during the reporting period.

Performance Timeframes

A measure's performance timeframe is defined in the measure's description and is distinct from the reporting frequency requirements defined in the measure's instructions. The performance timeframe, unique to each measure, outlines the timeframe in which the clinical action described in the numerator may be completed.

For example, Measure #110 (NQF 0041): Preventive Care and Screening: Influenza Immunization measures how many patients aged six months and older that were seen for a visit between October 1 and March 31 received an influenza immunization or reported previous receipt of an influenza immunization.

Although Quality is reported on the calendar year (Jan–Dec), flu season runs from October to March. To account for this discrepancy, the performance timeframe requires that in a given reporting year, the last half of the previous year's flu season (Jan–Mar) and the first half of the current year's flu season (Oct–Dec) are included in the measure's calculation.

For reference, the 2018 Measure specifications and supporting documentation can be downloaded from the QPP website.

Types of Measures

Measures can be used to evaluate the structure, process, and outcomes of care.

Structural quality measures include staff certifications, accreditation, and whether a practice or facility has the information technology in place to monitor and report care for patients. Structural measures are often thought of as minimum standards and necessary qualifications, but are not sufficient to ensure quality of care.

Process quality measures focus on steps that should be followed to provide evidence of quality care. There should be a scientific basis for believing that the process, when executed well, will increase the probability of achieving a desired outcome. Immunization rates and mammography screening rates are examples of process measures. Most measures of patient experience of care are process measures, such as whether a doctor explains tests and treatments in a way the patient can understand.

Outcome quality measures are the ultimate measurement of quality. They examine whether the outcomes for a population of patients are better, the same, or worse than expected for comparable patients. Commonly tracked outcome measures include surgical site infection rates, mortality rates, and rates of hospital readmission within a defined time. Outcome measures better reflect the totality of care provided, not just component processes and procedures.

High Priority quality measures are new to the MIPS program and are defined by CMS as an outcome, appropriate use, patient safety, efficiency, patient experience, or care coordination quality measures. If you've been paying attention, High Priority measures correlate to the NQS domains.

Cross-Cutting quality measures are any measures that are broadly applicable across multiple clinical settings and individual MIPS-eligible clinicians or groups within a variety of specialties.

Availability of Measures

Not all quality measures are available under each Quality reporting option. Of the 300+ individual measures included in the 2018 performance year, only a subset is available for each reporting method. In Table 3-1, there are 74 measures to choose from if the provider reports via claims. The subset for EHR-based reporting totals 53 different measures and those who choose this option can meet the requirements for multiple quality programs by reporting only once. With the alignment of quality measures across CMS quality reporting programs, some measures from the EHR Incentive Program may have been updated or modified during their NQF endorsement process. This may result in different measurement titles, number versions, or NQS domains from the corresponding Quality specification sheets.

TABLE 3-1. Measures Available by Reporting Method

Reporting Method	Available Measures to Report
Claims	74
Registry	243
EHR	53
Web Interface	15
QCDR	Varies by QCDR

Measure Selection Strategy

Because the availability of measures varies widely based on the reporting method, having a long-term strategy in place is crucial. It would be a shame to track a set of measures only to later discover they cannot be reported using your preferred method. By the same token, you would not want to decide on a particular method for reporting to later find that the available measures to report are not applicable to your specialty.

A smart start would begin by reviewing the Quality measures list to determine which ones best apply to the clinician and to the practice.

One of the best ways to find out which measures work for a clinician or practice is to spend some time searching for them on the Quality page of the QPP website. It is here that you can search by keyword and filter by measures that are considered high priority, as well as by data submission method and specialty measure set (Figure 3-3).

There are questions you may want answers to before selecting the right path to report quality data:

- Does your practice have an EHR? If so, do you know the quality measures that it is capable of capturing data for? And are at least six of those measures relevant to the clinician or clinicians in the practice?
- Are you a specialty provider? If so, does your specialty society recommend a particular registry or QCDR? Sometimes being a member of a specialty organization allows for participants to take advantage of member discounts.

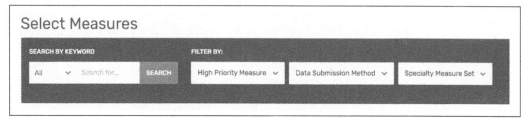

FIGURE 3-3. Searching for Measures on QPP

- Are there more than 25 clinicians in your practice? Are you a multi-specialty practice? If so, you may want to select the CMS Web Interface method of reporting.

And lastly, if none of the above applies to you, or leads you to a direct answer, you may want to consider claims-based reporting.

At minimum, consider these factors when selecting measures for reporting:
- Clinical conditions usually treated
- Types of care typically provided (e.g., preventive, chronic, acute)
- Settings where care is usually delivered (e.g., office, Emergency Department (ED), surgical suite)
- The quality measures your EHR is capable of tracking
- Quality improvement goals for the current year
- Reporting methods available for your selected measures
- Time/hours you want staff to dedicate to tracking measures
- Services most frequently provided to patients

Once possible measures have been selected, review the specification sheets for each (available on the QPP website) to make sure you understand each measure's reporting criteria. Specifically, review each measure's denominator coding to determine which patients may be eligible for the selected quality measures.

Next, start thinking about submission type.

Selecting the optimal measures and submission methods for your organization needs to be a cornerstone of your MIPS strategy.

It will be imperative that the six measures that a clinician chooses to report are relevant to his or her medical specialty and truly represent the quality of care provided to each patient. In many cases, a majority of the six measures could be specialty specific and the others could be cross-cutting measures. Cross-cutting measures are defined as relevant regardless of specialty, so this would translate into measuring something such as tobacco screening and cessation, screening for unhealthy alcohol use, or asking patients if they have had their flu shot.

Additionally, outcome and high priority measures are scored with more weight than other types of measures (e.g., a process or structural measure) and are thought of as the "golden child" of measure options because they show a patient's health outcome after a clinical action was taken. Remember, a process measure might quantify the rates of immunizations, screenings, or counseling, while a structural measure might track the amount of time spent with a patient or that a recall system is in place.

When deciding on specialty specific measures, keep an eye out for outcome measures—they may earn you more points.

Another way to find measures that are relevant to your specialty is by looking at CMS's Specialty Measure sets. There are 30 sets in total and all but three sets include six or more measures.

If the measure set contains fewer than six measures, MIPS-eligible clinicians will be required to report all available measures within the set. If the measure set contains six or more measures, MIPS-eligible clinicians will be required to report at least six measures within the set.

Regardless of the number of measures that are contained in the measure set, MIPS-eligible clinicians reporting on a measure set will be required to report at least one outcome measure or, if no outcome measures are available in the measure set, the MIPS-eligible clinician will report another high priority measure (e.g., appropriate use, patient safety, efficiency, patient experience, and care coordination measures) within the measure set in lieu of an outcome measure. MIPS-eligible clinicians may choose to report measures in addition to those contained in the specialty measure set.

The Specialty Sets included in MIPS are:

1. Allergy/Immunology—14 measures
2. Anesthesiology—9 measures
3. Cardiology—20 measures
4. Dermatology—11 measures
5. Diagnostic Radiology—14 measures
6. **Electrophysiology Cardiac Specialist—3 measures**
7. Emergency Medicine—15 measures
8. Gastroenterology—16 measures
9. General Oncology—19 measures
10. General Practice/Family Medicine—55 measures
11. General Surgery—14 measures
12. Hospitalists—13 measures
13. Internal Medicine—37 measures
14. **Interventional Radiology—4 measures**
15. Mental/Behavioral Health—25 measures
16. Neurology—26 measures
17. Obstetrics/Gynecology—24 measures

18. Ophthalmology—21 measures
19. Orthopedic Surgery—21 measures
20. Otolaryngology—18 measures
21. Pathology—8 measures
22. Pediatrics—18 measures
23. Physical Medicine—15 measures
24. Plastic Surgery—11 measures
25. Preventive Medicine—17 measures
26. **Radiation Oncology—4 measures**
27. Rheumatology—13 measures
28. Thoracic Surgery—15 measures
29. Urology—12 measures
30. Vascular Surgery–15 measures

As an example, the Dermatology Specialty Set includes the following 11 quality measures (see Table 3-2).

TABLE 3-2. Specialty Set for Dermatology

Quality ID#	Measure Name	Description
265	Biopsy Follow-Up	Percentage of new patients whose biopsy results have been reviewed and communicated to the primary care/referring physician and patient by the performing physician
374	Closing the Referral Loop: Receipt of Specialist Report	Percentage of patients with referrals, regardless of age, for which the referring provider receives a report from the provider to whom the patient was referred
130	Documentation of Current Medications in the Medical Record	Percentage of visits for patients aged 18 years and older for which the eligible professional attests to documenting a list of current medications using all immediate resources available on the date of the encounter (This list must include ALL known prescriptions, over-the-counters, herbals, and vitamin/mineral/dietary (nutritional) supplements AND must contain the medications' name, dosage, frequency, and route of administration.)
137	Melanoma: Continuity of Care—Recall System	Percentage of patients, regardless of age, with a current diagnosis of melanoma or a history of melanoma whose information was entered, at least once within a 12-month period, into a recall system that includes: • A target date for the next complete physical skin exam, AND • A process to follow up with patients who either did not make an appointment within the specified timeframe or who missed a scheduled appointment
138	Melanoma: Coordination of Care	Percentage of patient visits, regardless of age, with a new occurrence of melanoma who have a treatment plan documented in the chart that was communicated to the physician(s) providing continuing care within one month of diagnosis

(continued on next page)

TABLE 3-2. Specialty Set for Dermatology (continued)

Quality ID#	Measure Name	Description
224	Melanoma: Overutilization of Imaging Studies in Melanoma	Percentage of patients, regardless of age, with a current diagnosis of Stage O through IIC melanoma or a history of melanoma of any stage, without signs or symptoms suggesting systemic spread, seen for an office visit during the one-year measurement period, for whom no diagnostic imaging studies were ordered
317	Preventive Care and Screening: Screening for High Blood Pressure and Follow-up Documented	Percentage of patients aged 18 years and older seen during the reporting period who were screened for high blood pressure AND a recommended follow-up plan is documented based on the current blood pressure (BP) reading as indicated
226	Preventive Care and Screening: Tobacco Use: Screening and Cessation Intervention	Percentage of patients aged 18 years and older who were screened for tobacco use one or more times within 24 months AND who received cessation counseling intervention if identified as a tobacco user
410	Psoriasis: Clinical Response to Oral Systemic or Biologic Medications	Percentage of psoriasis patients receiving oral systemic or biologic therapy who meet minimal physician-or patient-reported disease activity levels. It is implied that establishment and maintenance of an established minimum level of disease control as measured by physician-and/or patient-reported outcomes will increase patient satisfaction with and adherence to treatment
402	Tobacco Use and Help with Quitting Among Adolescents	The percentage of adolescents 12 to 20 years of age with a primary care visit during the measurement year for whom tobacco use status was documented and received help with quitting if identified as a tobacco user
337	Tuberculosis (TB) Prevention for Psoriasis, Psoriatic Arthritis, and Rheumatoid Arthritis Patients on a Biological Immune Response	Percentage of patients whose providers are ensuring active tuberculosis prevention either through yearly negative standard tuberculosis screening tests or are reviewing the patient's history to determine if they have had appropriate management for a recent or prior positive test

MIPS-eligible clinicians or groups are expected to report on applicable measures, where "applicable" is defined as measures relevant to a particular MIPS-eligible clinician's services or care rendered. MIPS-eligible clinicians can refer to the measures' specifications to verify which measures are applicable. Not all measures in each Specialty Measure Set will be applicable to all clinicians in a given specialty. If the set includes fewer than six applicable measures, the eligible clinician should only report the measures that are applicable.

In most cases, eligible clinicians will want to review and select up to six measures that best fit their practice, making sure to include at least one outcome measure, or a high priority measure if an outcome measure is not available.

Submission Methods Available

It will also be important to understand the method by which the clinician or practice plans to submit the measure data, as reporting requirements may vary slightly, depending on the method.

Claims-Based Reporting:

With claims-based reporting, measures are tied to clinical practice reported on *claims* with ICD-10, CPT, HCPCS, and G-codes that link to measures for covered services under the Medicare Part B Physician Fee Schedule. These codes identify which patients should be added toward the denominator/numerator of a quality measure.

Data submission is the responsibility of the eligible clinician or the billing company.

The following example reports the Breast Cancer Resection Pathology Reporting measure on a claim (Figure 3-4). For the measure's denominator, the diagnosis for breast cancer is indicated in field 21 of the form, and the

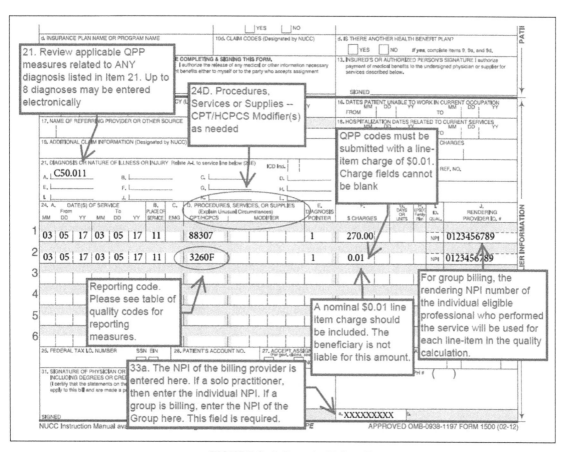

FIGURE 3-4. Sample Claims Form

CPT code for tissue exam by pathologist in line 1 of field 24. For the measure's numerator, the quality measure code is reported in line 2 to indicate performance was met.

Notice that in order for quality data codes to be accepted by CMS, they need to have a nominal charge associated with them. A nominal charge can be as low as $0.01.

If you bill $0.00 for a quality data code line item, you'll get a Remittance Advice (RA)/Explanation of Benefits (EOB) with the N620 code, which informs you that CMS acknowledges your coding effort, but also that there was an error, or your billing entry wasn't submitted correctly.

N620 shows that a procedure isn't payable unless non-payable reporting codes and the right modifiers are submitted. On the Remittance Advice, the N620 code will state: *This procedure code is for quality reporting/informational purposes only.*

Advantages of Claims-Based Reporting:

1. You are in control of your own data from completion to submission.
2. You can develop a self-auditing process to meet your clinic's specific needs.
3. There are no additional costs to report.
4. The 60 percent data completeness requirement is in regards to Medicare patients only, not all insurance payers for the 2018 program year.
5. It's an ideal reporting option for a solo practitioner, a smaller practice, or if Medicare is a minimal portion of your payer mix.

Disadvantages of Claims-Based Reporting:

1. If the Medicare Administrative Contractor (MAC) denies payment for all the billable services on your claim, the quality data codes will not be included in your MIPS analysis, so your data will not count toward your MIPS participation.
2. If you correct a denied claim and it gets paid through an adjustment, re-opening, or the appeals process by the MAC with accurate codes that match the measure's denominator, then any of the quality data codes that apply and align with the numerator should also be included on your corrected claim.
3. You cannot resubmit claims only to add or correct quality data codes. However, you can resubmit claims with *only* quality data codes on them with a $0.00 or $0.01 total dollar amount to the MAC.
4. You should have someone in the clinic who will own this project, as he will need to consistently add quality data codes to claims, keep records of the percent complete, and understand Quality for MIPS.

5. The workload could be significant if a large percent of your patients are insured through Medicare or you work in a large clinic.
6. Earning bonus points for submitting additional High Priority measures is not available for this reporting method.
7. Earning bonus points for electronic reporting is not available for this reporting method.
8. There is no internal automated check and balance system; if a claim is missing quality data codes, you cannot resubmit the claim to fix it.

For 2018, Registry-, EHR-, and QCDR-based reporting require 60 percent of all eligible data, for *all* insurance payers for each measure to qualify for the maximum achievement scores.

Registry-Based:

With registry-based reporting, the eligible clinician or group practice submits the data electronically to the registry, that then captures and stores the measure related data. The registry is then responsible for aggregating the submitted data, compiling it into a digital format, and submitting it directly to CMS on behalf of eligible clinicians. Registries provide CMS with calculated reporting and performance rates at the end of the reporting period. In order to be qualified as a registry vendor, each must annually pass stringent reporting method criteria.

Many registries can interface directly with your EHR, so as you document patient data within your EHR, the numerator and denominator information populate a report so you can easily review your performance.

Some, but not all, registries have built-in benchmark data within their dashboards, so you can see right away if your performance on each measure is above or below the target. For those that do not have it build in, you would have to cross-reference published CMS's benchmarks.

Advantages of Registry-Based Reporting:

1. With an EHR integration, data collection for all eligible patients is automatically enforced.
2. Quality data submission is done for you.
3. There is reduced administrative burden on billing and reporting staff.
4. Many quality measures are eligible for bonus points for reporting additional High Priority measures.
5. In many cases, reporting through a registry qualifies for bonus points for end-to-end electronic reporting.
6. Real-time reports identify whether or not you are on track.
7. Your Quality score is clearly communicated.

For 2018, Registry-, EHR-, and QCDR-based reporting require 60 percent of all eligible data, for *all* insurance payers for each measure to qualify for the maximum achievement scores.

Disadvantages of Registry-Based Reporting:

1. There is a cost involved, typically $300 per eligible clinician.
2. Unlike claims-based reporting, the 60 percent data completeness requirement applies to *all* payers for the 2018 program year.

QCDR-Based:

A qualified clinical data registry (QCDR) is "an organized system that uses observational study methods to collect uniform data (clinical and other) to evaluate specified outcomes for a population defined by a particular disease, condition, or exposure, and that serves one or more predetermined scientific, clinical, or policy purposes."

The QCDR reporting option is different from a qualified registry because it allows clinicians to report quality measures that are outside of the QPP measure list.

Generally speaking, "QCDR measures" are tailored toward specialists, which can contribute to more meaningful, quality reporting. For example, gastroenterologists can report clinically relevant information about colonoscopies or upper GI endoscopies through the GIQuiC QCDR; urologists can report clinically relevant information about prostate cancer or urinary incontinence through the AQUA QCDR; dermatologists can report clinically relevant information about psoriasis, basal cell carcinomas, or biopsy reports through the DataDerm QCDR.

To be eligible for reporting, each "QCDR measure" must be first approved by CMS.

Each year, CMS will announce the QCDRs that have been approved to report quality measure data to CMS on behalf of eligible clinicians.

Many QCDRs (but not all) can also integrate with EHRs. If this is true for you, it may decrease your documentation burden because your QCDR can capture data taken directly from your daily workflow to include in your electronic submission to CMS.

Advantages of QCDR-Based Reporting:

1. For QCDRs that integrate directly with your EHR, the data collection for all eligible patients is automatically ingested.
2. QCDRs may offer more specialty-specific quality measures that could be more applicable to the care you provide.
3. Quality data submission is done for you.
4. There is a reduced administrative burden on billing and reporting staff.
5. If QCDR is interfaced with your EHR, it may be eligible for bonus points for end-to-end electronic reporting.
6. Real-time reports identify whether or not you are on track.

7. There are several QCDR-related Improvement Activities that can be used to earn points in that MIPS category.
8. One QCDR-related Improvement Activity (ID # IA_AHE_2) is also eligible for a bonus in the ACI category for clinicians who have met the Base Score requirements.
9. CMS finalized a 5% bonus in the ACI category for reporting to one or more public health or clinical data registries, including QCDRs, beyond the immunization registry reporting measure.

Disadvantages of QCDR-Based Reporting:

1. There is a cost involved, typically $300 per eligible clinician.
2. The 60 percent data completeness requirement applies to *all* payers for the 2018 program year.
3. Participating in a QCDR may take time to implement, especially if it requires integrating or interfacing with your EHR.
4. This reporting is not eligible for bonus points for reporting additional High Priority measures.

EHR-Based Reporting:

With EHR-based reporting, compiling quality measure data relies upon information routinely collected during the course of providing clinical care and that is documented directly within the clinician's EHR.

Generally speaking, every certified EHR can track a minimum of nine electronic clinical quality measures (eCQMs), although many can track all of the approved eCQMs included in the program.

Some EHRs are capable of submitting quality data directly to CMS on behalf of eligible clinicians. However, for the most part, the onus is on the clinician or group to export a specific type of digital file, called a QRDA III, which then must be imported into Quality Net for official submission.

Using the EHR to report quality measures can offer higher scores because the benchmarks tend to be more favorable for this method and using the structured format of the system creates more opportunities to earn bonus points.

Advantages of EHR-Based Reporting:

1. Data collection occurs concurrently while documenting routine clinical care within the EHR.
2. Many EHRs have built-in benchmark and MIPS scoring data to easily track your performance.
3. Measures qualify for the end-to-end electronic reporting bonus.
4. This reporting is eligible for bonus points when you report additional High Priority measures.

5. There is no additional cost from the EHR vendor to report in this manner.

Disadvantages of EHR-Based Reporting:

1. The EHR export/Quality Net import process can be challenging. It requires the EHR to export a properly formatted QRDA type III report, and for the user to both obtain access and security roles for Quality Net, and go through a data validation process before officially submitting to CMS.
2. The 60 percent data completeness requirement applies to *all* payers for the 2018 program year.

Web Interface Reporting:

The CMS Web Interface reporting option is only available to groups with 25 or more eligible clinicians, as defined by taxpayer identification number (TIN). This method is not recommended for newly formed group practices or group practices that do not provide primary care services.

The Web Interface tracks 15 pre-selected quality measures (Table 3-3). *All* of them, regardless of the specialty type of the group, must be reported for the first 248 consecutively ranked beneficiaries in the sample for each measure or module. If fewer than 248 beneficiaries are assigned to the group, the group must report on 100% of the assigned beneficiaries. If a group has no assigned patients, then the group or individuals within the group need to select another mechanism to submit data to MIPS.

Groups that wish to report through this method must register with CMS between April 1 and June 30 of the reporting year.

The reported data must include sampling requirements for Medicare Part B patients.

The performance period is the entire calendar year, January 1 to December 31, of the performance year.

Advantages of Web Interface-Based Reporting:
1. The Web Interface only accepts Medicare patient quality data.
2. There is reduced administrative burden for larger groups.
3. The risk of data entry errors is minimized.

Disadvantages of Web Interface-Based Reporting:
1. Measures are geared more toward primary care, so specialists may not be well represented by the quality measures.

CAHPS for MIPS:

A registered group of two or more MIPS-eligible clinicians may elect to participate in the "CAHPS for MIPS" Survey. (Table 3-4 Summary Survey Measures included in CAHPS for MIPS)

TABLE 3-3. Web Interface Measures

Web Interface Measure Number	Measure Title	Alternative Measure Identifiers: Quality, QCO, NQF, CMS (For reference only)
Care Coordination/Patient Safety (CARE) Measures 2 Measures—Individually Sampled)		
CARE-1	Medication Reconciliation Post Discharge	Quality ID # 46 ACO 12 NQF 0097
CARE-2	Falls: Screening for Future Fall Risk	Quality ID #318 Web Interface Only ACO 13 NQF 0101 CMS 139v6
Diabetes Composite (Single Composite Consisting of Two Measures) Composite: All or Nothing Scoring		
DM-2	Composite (All or Nothing Scoring): Diabetes: Hemoglobin A1c (HbA1c) Poor Control (>9%)	Quality ID #1 ACO 27 NQF 0059 CMS 122v6
DM-7	Composite (All or Nothing Scoring): Diabetes: Eye Exam	Quality ID #117 ACO 41 NQF 0055 CMS131v6
Hypertension (HTN) Disease Measure		
HTN-2	Controlling High Blood Pressure	Quality ID #236 ACO 28 NQF 0018 CMS 165v6
Ischemic Vascular Disease (IVD) Measure		
IVD-2	Ischemic Vascular Disease (IVD): Use of Aspirin or Another Antiplatelet	Quality ID #204 ACO 30 NQF 0068 CMS 164v6
Mental Health (MH) Disease Measure		
MH-1	Depression Remission at 12 Months	Quality ID #370 (Registry Only ACO 40 NQF 0710 CMS 159v6
Preventive (PREV) Care Measures (8 Measures—Individually Sampled)		
PREV-5	Breast Cancer Screening	Quality ID #112 ACO 20 NQF 2372 CMS 125v6

(continued on next page)

TABLE 3-3. Web Interface Measures (continued)

Web Interface Measure Number	Measure Title	Alternative Measure Identifiers: Quality, QCO, NQF, CMS (For reference only)
PREV-6	Colorectal Cancer Screening	Quality ID #113 ACO 19 NQF 0034 CMS 130v6
PREV-7	Preventive Care and Screening: Influenza Immunization	Quality ID #110 ACO 14 NQF 0041 CMS 147v7
PREV-8	Pneumonia Vaccination Status for Older Adults	Quality ID #111 ACO 15 NQF 0043 CMS 127v6
PREV-9	Preventive Care and Screening: Body Mass Index (BMI) Screening and Follow-Up Plan	Quality ID #128 ACO 16 NQF 0421 CMS 69v6
PREV-10	Preventive Care and Screening: Tobacco Use: Screening and Cessation Intervention	Quality ID #226 ACO 17 NQF 0028 CMS 138v6
PREV-12	Preventive Care and Screening: Screening for Depression and Follow-Up Plan	Quality ID #134 ACO 18 NQF 0418 CMS2v6
PREV-13	Statin Therapy for the Prevention and Treatment of Cardiovascular Disease	Quality ID #438 Registry Only ACO 42 CMS 347v1

Reporting "CAHPS for MIPS" equates to one patient experience survey, as well as a "patient experience" measure. Please note that a "patient experience" measure replaces the need for an outcome measure if there are no applicable outcome measures available to fit the practice.

Groups may report on any five measures within MIPS plus the "CAPHS for MIPS" survey to achieve the six-measure threshold (Table 3-4).

Groups that choose the "CAHPS for MIPS" survey option must use a CMS-approved vendor and have them report the group's results to CMS on their behalf.

To report on five other MIPS measures, the group must use one of the other submission methods. The survey must be administered from November to February. The data must include sampling requirements for Medicare Part B patients. The performance period is the entire calendar year, January 1 to December 31, of the performance year.

TABLE 3-4. Summary Survey Measures included in CAHPS for MIPS

Summary Survey Measure	Included in the CAHPS for MIPS Survey?	Included in CAHPS for MIPS Scoring?
Getting Timely Care, Appointments, and Information	Yes	Yes
How Well Providers Communicate	Yes	Yes
Patient's Rating of Provider	Yes	Yes
Health Promotion & Education	Yes	Yes
Shared Decision Making	Yes	Yes
Stewardship of Patient Resources	Yes	Yes
Courteous and Helpful Office Staff	Yes	Yes
Care Coordination	Yes	Yes
Health Status and Functional Status	Yes	No
Access to Specialists	Yes	No

Advantages of CAHPS for MIPS-Based Reporting:

1. Patients' perceptions of their care are reflections of the doctor-patient relationship and include holistic aspects of healing and emotional well-being. If we care about the experience of our patients, why shouldn't we measure it and strive to improve our performance?
2. Practices that have better engagement with patients may encourage greater adherence to clinical standards of care and follow-up. Patients who are more satisfied with a practice may be more likely to return for visits and follow the recommendations of the clinicians that they trust.
3. Practices with better patient experience scores could indicate that they have stronger teamwork, organizational leadership, and commitment to improvement. These are all characteristics that could be associated with better quality measures and patient experience scores.

Disadvantages of CAHPS for MIPS-Based Reporting:

1. It is impossible to control the survey results.
2. Faced with penalties for low patient satisfaction scores, physicians could avoid caring for patients who may be more challenging to treat and perceived to be difficult to please. This includes underserved minorities, those with lower socioeconomic status, and/or those with mental health concerns.
3. Patient experience measures are based on patients' expectation of care as opposed to objective measures of experience.
4. The surveys are voluntary, relatively long, and are often answered many weeks after the experience. There may be selection and recall bias in the responses of those with very positive or negative experiences.

Regardless of the path you choose, you will want to ensure that processes are in place to capture and report quality data as early in the year as feasibly possible, to be confident that you'll meet the data completeness criteria.

Data Completeness Requirements

Once you've selected the quality measures you wish to track, as well as a reporting method, you'll want to make sure you capture enough information for each measure to meet CMS' data completeness requirements. (Table 3-5 Data Completeness Requirements by Submission Mechanism)

Each submission method, clinician type, submission criteria, and data completeness requirement is outlined in Table 3-5.

I'll note here, a few factors worth paying attention to:

- Claims-based reporting is only available to clinicians reporting as individuals.
- QCDR-, Registry-, and EHR-based reporting requires reporting on patients across all payers, while other methods require reporting just on Medicare Part B patients.
- Web Interface-based reporting is only available to groups with 25 or more clinicians.

CMS-Calculated Population-Based Measures

This section applies to groups that are *not* considered a "small practice." CMS defines a small practice as 15 or fewer eligible clinicians and they use claims data from Sept. 1, 2016 to Aug. 31, 2017, plus a 30-day claims run out to determine which practices will be deemed "small" for the 2018 program year.

If you are in a group of 16 or more eligible clinicians, this section is for you. All others can skip ahead.

It is important to know that there are three population-based quality measures that CMS tracks that offer clinicians minimal control over their outcomes. Thankfully for now, only one of these population-based measures will be tied to a MIPS score, and even then, only under certain conditions.

These population-based quality measures include:

1. CMS-1: Acute Composite Measure, which tracks the three following measures:
   a. Bacterial Pneumonia (NQF 0279)
      i. This measure is used to assess the number of admissions with a principal diagnosis of bacterial pneumonia per 1,000 population, ages 18 years and older. It excludes sickle cell or hemoglobin-S admissions, other indications of immunocompromised state admissions, obstetric admissions, and transfers from other institutions.

TABLE 3-5. Data Completeness Requirements by Submission Mechanism

Performance Period	Clinician Type	Submission Mechanism	Submission Criteria	Data Completeness
Jan 1–Dec 31	Individual MIPS-Eligible Clinicians	Part B Claims	Report at least six measures including one outcome measure, or if an outcome measure is not available, report another high priority measure; if less than six measures apply, then report on each measure that is applicable. Individual MIPS-eligible clinicians would have to select their measures from either the set of all MIPS measures listed or referenced, or one of the specialty measure sets listed in, the applicable final rule.	Sixty percent of individual MIPS-eligible clinician's Medicare Part B patients for the performance period
Jan 1–Dec 31	Individual MIPS-Eligible Clinicians, Groups	QCDR, Registry, and EHR	Report at least six measures including one outcome measure, or if an outcome measure is not available, report another high priority measure; if less than six measures apply, then report on each measure that is applicable. Individual MIPS-eligible clinicians, or groups would have to select their measures from either the set of all MIPS measures listed or referenced, or one of the specialty measure sets listed in the applicable final rule.	Sixty percent of individual MIPS-eligible clinician's or group's patients across all payers for the performance period
Jan 1–Dec 31	Groups	CMS Web Interface	Report on all measures included in the CMS Web Interface; AND populate data fields for the first 248 consecutively ranked and assigned Medicare beneficiaries in the order in which they appear in the group's sample for each module/measure. If the pool of eligible assigned beneficiaries is less than 248, then the group would report on 100 percent of assigned beneficiaries.	Sampling requirements for the group's Medicare Part B patients
Jan 1–Dec 31	Groups	CAHPS for MIPS Survey	CMS-approved survey vendor would need to be paired with another reporting mechanism to ensure the minimum number of measures is reported. CAHPS for MIPS survey would fulfill the requirement for one patient experience measure towards the MIPS quality data submission criteria. CAHPS for MIPS survey would only count for one measure under the quality performance category.	Sampling requirements for the group's Medicare Part B patients

    b. Urinary Tract Infections (NQF 0281)

       i. This measure is used to assess the number of admissions for urinary tract infection per 100,000 population.

    c. Dehydration (NQF 0280)

       i. This measure is used to assess the number of admissions for dehydration per 100,000 population.

2. CMS-2: Chronic Composite Measure, which tracks a total of six measures, outlined below:

    a. Diabetes (NQF 0274, 0272, 0285, 0638)

      i. NQF 0274: This measure is used to assess the number of admissions for long-term diabetes complications per 100,000 population.

      ii. NQF 0272: This measure assesses the number of admissions for diabetes short-term complications per 100,000 population.

      iii. NQF 0285: This measure is used to assess the number of admissions for lower-extremity amputation among patients with diabetes per 100,000 population.

      iv. NQF 0638: This measure assesses the number of admissions for uncontrolled diabetes among patients with diabetes per 100,000 population.

  b. Chronic Obstructive Pulmonary Disease or Asthma (NQF 0275)

      i. This measure assesses Admissions of a principal diagnosis of chronic obstructive pulmonary disease (COPD) or asthma per 1,000 population, ages 40 years and older. It excludes obstetric admissions and transfers from other institutions.

  c. Heart Failure (NQF 0277)

      i. This measure assesses admissions with a principal diagnosis of heart failure per 100,000 population, ages 18 years and older.

3. CMS-3: All-Cause Hospital Readmissions Measure

  a. The 30-day all-cause readmission measure is a risk-standardized readmission rate for beneficiaries aged 65 or older who were hospitalized at a short-stay acute care hospital and experienced an unplanned readmission for any cause to an acute care hospital within 30 days of discharge.

Originally, MIPS-eligible clinicians were set to be evaluated on their performance on each of these measures in addition to the six required quality measures. However, CMS did a reliability analysis in 2016 that indicated the first two of these measures are not reliable indicators for solo clinicians or practices with fewer than 16 clinicians. Since further testing and enhancements will be required, only the All-Cause Hospital Readmission measure will be incorporated into the MIPS scores for groups of 16 or more eligible clinicians who have beneficiaries attributed to them and that meet the minimum case size requirement. CMS believes this measure encourages care coordination.

Eligible clinicians in groups with 16 or more clinicians and at least 200 cases would be evaluated on their performance on the All-Cause Hospital Readmission measure, in addition to the six required quality measures.

If the case minimum of 200 cases has not been met, CMS will not score this measure. The MIPS-eligible clinicians associated with groups of 16 or more will not receive a zero for this measure and this measure will not apply to the MIPS-eligible clinician's quality performance category score.

Be warned that CMS will continue to calculate all three of these measures for all MIPS-eligible clinicians and provide feedback for informational purposes as part of the MIPS feedback that is published each July after the previous year's reporting.

Additionally, CMS intends to incorporate a clinical risk adjustment as soon as feasible to the composite measures and continue to research ways to develop and use other population-based measures for the MIPS program that could be applied to greater numbers of MIPS-eligible clinicians going forward.

Benchmarking Providers

When quality measure data is submitted, CMS compares each clinician's performance results to benchmarks from the prior year, leaving room to make some adjustments based on patient risk factors and the clinician's location.

Benchmarking is the process of comparing a practice's performance with an external standard. It is an important tool that CMS uses to motivate clinicians and practices to engage in improvement work and to help members of a practice understand where their performance falls in comparison to other providers. Benchmarking can stimulate healthy competition, as well as help members of a practice reflect more effectively on their own performance.

Each year, CMS will analyze the performance rates submitted for each quality measure included in the program and will create individual benchmarks for each as well. Ultimately, the prior year's performance is used to set the stage for the current year's benchmark, which helps determine a clinician's score for each quality measure.

Keep in mind that the same measure may have up to three different benchmarks, depending on the number of ways in which data may be reported for that measure. For some measures, data can be reported three different ways (e.g., by claims, EHR, or registry), whereas some measures require data to be reported in one specified manner (e.g., registry only).

If a clinician or practice wants to predict their Quality score, it is imperative to know and understand the benchmarks tied to the selected measures. A sample measure's benchmark data is outlined below. Through this, one can begin to forecast a score. For example, if a clinician were to submit a performance rate of 82 percent for this sample measure, she would earn somewhere between 9.0 to 9.9 points in the Quality category. If she does this for five more measures, she can start to work her way up to the maximum 60 points.

Take, for example, the measure for "Tobacco Use Screening and Cessation Intervention," which requires physicians to screen adult patients

Keep in mind that the same measure may have up to three different benchmarks, depending on the number of ways in which data may be reported for that measure. For some measures, data can be reported three different ways (e.g., by claims, EHR, or registry), whereas some measures require data to be reported in one specified manner (e.g., registry only).

for tobacco use every 24 months and intervene if the patient identifies as a tobacco user (Table 3-6). For this measure, a physician or group may report by administrative claims, EHR, or registry. As demonstrated in Table 3-6, the benchmarks for this measure vary significantly based on the data submission method.

TABLE 3-6. Benchmark Differences by Submission Method Example

Tobacco Use: Screening and Cessation Intervention									
Submission Method	Decile 3	Decile 4	Decile 5	Decile 6	Decile 7	Decile 8	Decile 9	Decile 10	Topped Out
Claims	95.60–97.85	99.26–99.99	–	–	–	–	–	100	Y
EHR	72.59–81.59	86.60–86.68	86.69–90.15	90.16–92.64	92.65–94.67	94.68–96.58	96.59–98.51	≥98.52	N
Registry/QCDR	76.67–85.53	85.54–89.53	89.88–92.85	92.86–95.14	95.15–97.21	97.22–99.10	99.11–99.99	100	N

With the introduction of different benchmarks, CMS has increased the analytical complexity of selecting the optimal set of measures and reporting methods for MIPS. With the financial and reputational impacts of MIPS, it is important to ensure you are making decisions that will best position your organization for success.

CMS has a way of making this extra complicated. They have established distinct benchmarks for different reporting methods. This means a performance rate of 82 percent may earn the clinician 9.5 points if reporting via registry, but may only earn the clinician 5.9 points if reporting via claims, or eight points if reporting via EHR.

For each measure that has more than one reporting option, the benchmark values vary, in many cases significantly, between the submission methods.

CMS determines each measure's benchmark based on the reporting mechanism. Therefore, the following will have separate benchmarks:

- EHRs
- Qualified Clinical Data Registry and other registries
- CMS Web Interface
- Administrative claims measures
- Consumer Assessment of Healthcare Providers and Systems (CAHPS) survey for MIPS

If a benchmark is not available for a certain measure, then clinicians will automatically receive three points for submitting data on that measure.

If you report more than six quality measures, CMS will count the highest scoring six to determine your category score.

It can be a tricky balance to find the measures that are best suited for a clinician, that also have favorable benchmarks. And we haven't even reviewed Topped Out measures yet!

Topped Out Measures

And here we are. Let's take a closer look at Topped Out measures.

Physicians should look for meaningful quality measures that present a fair opportunity to score well relative to the established benchmarks. One indicator of such opportunity is whether a measure is "topped out"—meaning there is little difference between the worst and best performers on the measure. Once a measure tops out, it may be close to retirement, as there is no longer an opportunity for improvement in the performance it measures. That is, for these measures, overall performance is so high (near 100 percent) that CMS denotes that the measures are no longer meaningful to collect and report.

In order for CMS to issue a measure "topped out" status, the measure should:

- show statistically indistinguishable performance at the 75th and 90th percentiles; and
- also have a truncated coefficient of variation ≤0.10.

In plain English, all scores are relative: a score of 95 percent isn't worth much if 90 percent of physicians scored at 96 percent or above.

Each measure and its corresponding submission method must meet two criteria in order to be deemed "topped out."

Take, for example, the measure for "Tobacco Use Screening and Cessation Intervention," which requires physicians to screen adult patients for tobacco use every 24 months and intervene if the patient identifies as a tobacco user. For this measure, a physician or group may report by claims, EHR, or registry. As demonstrated in the table for Tobacco Use, the benchmarks for this measure vary significantly based on the data submission method.

In the Tobacco Use example, there are three submission methods available, but only one of them is considered topped out.

If a physician elects to report by claims, he or she could receive no more than five points on this measure if the physician or group failed to screen or intervene for a *single* tobacco user. By comparison, physicians and groups who report through their EHRs or through a registry would receive more points for less-than-perfect performance.

Not to go too far down the statistics rabbit hole, but when the majority of providers submit high performance rates for a particular method—and

If you report more than six quality measures, CMS will count the highest scoring six to determine your category score.

TABLE 3-7. 2018 Capped Measures

Measure Name	Measure ID	Measure Type	Topped Out for All Submission Mechanisms	Included in These Specialty Set(s)
Perioperative Care: Selection of Prophylactic Antibiotic—First OR Second Generation Cephalosporin	21	Process	Yes	General Surgery, Orthopedic Surgery, Otolaryngology, Thoracic Surgery, Plastic Surgery
Melanoma: Overutilization of Imaging Studies in Melanoma	224	Process	Yes	Dermatology
Perioperative Care: Venous Thromboembolism (VTE) Prophylaxis (When Indicated in ALL Patients)	23	Process	Yes	General Surgery, Orthopedic Surgery, Otolaryngology, Thoracic Surgery, Plastic Surgery
Image Confirmation of Successful Excision of Image-Localized Breast Lesion	262	Process	Yes	N/A

in this case, claims—the result is a higher mean. A higher mean indicates to CMS that the majority of providers who submitted this measure in this manner had a high level of success.

CMS then performs a calculation to identify the spread of data and identifies if there is a large concentration of high performers. If the median performance rate for a measure passes a certain threshold, CMS will reclassify it as topped out and apply a different scoring methodology.

Practically speaking, a measure's "topped out" status could lead you to report the same measure, but through a method that is not topped out, or select a new measure to report altogether, since the points available are limited. For example, you could report the Tobacco Use measure by registry instead of claims to gain access to higher points.

Thankfully, for MIPS performance year 2018, the majority of topped out quality measures are not scored differently than all other quality measures. For each set of benchmarks, CMS calculates the decile breaks for measure performance and assigns points based on which benchmark decile range the MIPS-eligible clinician's measure rate falls between.

Capping Topped Out Measures

For 2018, CMS will be capping Topped Out Measures. CMS will apply a special scoring cap of seven points to topped out measures. The cap will create incentives for clinicians to submit other measures for which they can improve and earn future improvement points (Table 3-7).

TABLE 3-8. Changes in Scoring Topped Out Measures Starting in the CY 2018 MIPS Performance Period

Scoring Policy	Measure 1 (topped out)	Measure 2 (topped out)	Measure 3 (topped out)	Measure 4 (topped out)	Measure 5 (not topped out)	Measure 6 (not topped out)	Quality Category Percent Score*
2017 MIPS Perf. Period Scoring	10 measure achievement points	10 measure achievement points	10 measure achievement points	4 measure achievement points (did not get max score)	10 measure achievement points	5 measure achievement points	49/60 = 81.67%
Capped Scoring Applied (2018 and Beyond)	7 measure achievement points	7 measure achievement points	7 measure achievement points	4 measure achievement points	10 measure achievement points	5 measure achievement points	40/60 = 66.67%
Notes	Topped out measures scored with seven-point measure achievement point cap. The cap does not impact score if the MIPS-eligible clinician is below the cap.				Still possible to earn maximum achievement points on the non-topped out measures.		

* This example would only apply to the six measures identified for the CY 2018 MIPS Performance Period. This example also excludes bonus points and improvement scoring.

CMS will apply the special scoring policy to the six selected measures for the 2018 MIPS performance period and 2020 MIPS payment year.

The six measures identified in Table 3-8 will receive a maximum of seven measure achievement points, provided that for the applicable submission mechanisms, the measure benchmarks are identified as topped out again in the benchmarks published for the 2018 MIPS performance period. Beginning with the 2021 MIPS payment year, measure benchmarks (except for measures in the CMS Web Interface) that are identified as topped out for two or more consecutive years will receive a maximum of seven measure achievement points in the second consecutive year they are identified as topped out, and beyond.

Any high priority measure that is topped out will still be eligible for bonus points. CMS believes incentives should remain to report high priority measures, even topped out measures, as additional reporting makes for a more comprehensive benchmark and can help confirm that the measure is truly topped out.

However, CMS will modify the benchmark methodology for topped out measures beginning with the 2018 performance period, provided that it is the second year the measure has been identified as topped out.

Although you may have a high-performance rate in a topped out measure, it will be significantly harder for you to earn high points for that measure.

As the tobacco cessation measure demonstrated, a measure may be topped out if reported in one way, but not others. Of the measures that may

The six measures identified in Table 3-8, 2018 Capped Measures, will receive a maximum of seven measure achievement points

be reported by Part B claims, nearly 60 percent are topped out. If a physician reports on one of these measures by claims, it will be difficult for her to earn even intermediate points if she falls short of 100 percent performance on that measure.

Nearly half of the measures reported by registry are topped out, while only 10 percent of the EHR-reported measures are topped out. Based on this metric alone, EHR reporting may present the greatest opportunity for physicians to earn higher points for quality measures.

It really depends on what options you have available to you via your EHR, a specialty-specific registry, or working with your biller to add Quality Data Codes (QDC) to claims.

Tracking your progress may take concentrated effort, depending on your method of reporting Quality data.

Registries interfaced with EHRs typically include benchmark data.

Registry, QCDR, and EHR-based reporting allow for more time to complete documentation and review results before submitting to CMS.

Claims-based reporters must add quality data codes to claims at the time of billing the encounter.

Claims-based reporters will have only one chance to get feedback on their progress—when CMS releases feedback reports, typically in July.

Quality Performance Category Scoring

Next, let's take a look at how CMS scores the Quality category. The maximum number of points available in the Quality category depends on the size of the practice as well as the method of submission. (Figure 3-5 Scoring the Quality Category through Claims, Registry, EHR, or QCDR)

For those who report via claims, registry, QCDR, or EHR, the total score could be:

- **60 points** for individuals or groups with complete reporting and where no readmission measure applies; or
- **70 points** for groups with complete reporting and where the readmission measure applies.

The points can be earned as shown in Figure 3.5.

To maximize one's quality component score, a physician must report individually or as part of a group, on a minimum of six measures, at least one of which must be an outcome measure.

To break this down further, clinicians would select six of the approximately 300 quality measures available, and report for a minimum of 90 days to earn an Achievement Score. Depending on your specialty and group size, you may also choose to report a specialty set or via the CMS Web Interface.

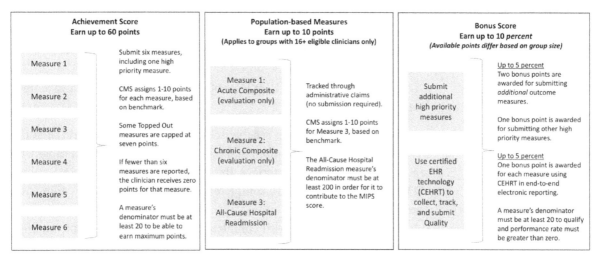

FIGURE 3-5. Scoring the Quality Category through Claims, Registry, EHR, or QCDR

For groups with at least 16 clinicians and a sufficient number of cases, the readmission measure will also be included in the score.

For each measure submitted for the 2018 performance year, clinicians will receive anywhere from three to 10 points based on their performance against the national benchmarks.

Zero points are earned for quality measures that are not submitted or that lack performance data.

There is a minimum case volume criteria needed to receive more than three points for each measure, so in some cases, choosing a longer reporting period can allow for higher points.

To maximize one's quality component score, a physician must report individually, or as part of a group, on a minimum of six measures, at least one of which must be an outcome measure. Under MIPS's predecessor, the Physician Quality Reporting System (PQRS), most physicians reported on a subset of their Medicare patients. With MIPS, however, a physician or group must report on at least 50% of their relevant patient population depending on their submission type.

Remember the benchmarking discussion? CMS collects all the measure data, has established performance benchmarks based on a prior period or the performance period, and then scores MIPS-eligible clinicians based on their performance relative to the benchmarks.

For both the 2017 and 2018 performance years, clinicians automatically receive three points for completing and submitting a measure, even if there is no benchmark and data completeness requirement is not met.

If a measure can be reliably scored against a benchmark, then a clinician can receive three to 10 points.

> To maximize one's quality component score, a physician must report individually or as part of a group, on a minimum of six measures, at least one of which must be an outcome measure.

If a measure can be reliably scored against a benchmark, then a clinician can receive three to 10 points.

Reliable score means the following:
- A benchmark exists.
- A clinician has sufficient case volume (≥20 cases for most measures; ≥200 cases for readmissions).
- Data completeness is met (at least 60 percent of possible data is submitted).

If a measure cannot be reliably scored against a benchmark, then the clinician will receive a maximum of three points (Figure 3-6). For those who report via the CMS Web Interface, the total score could be:
- **110 points** for groups with complete reporting and where no readmission measure applies; or
- **120 points** for groups with complete reporting and where the readmission measure applies.

The points can be earned as shown in Figure 3-6.

Each Quality measure is converted to points (1-10). Maximum points are available when data completeness criterion is met (percent of patients reported), the denominator is at least 20, and the performance is greater than the national benchmark.

Points will only be earned if the minimum number of measures is submitted. ECs who do not report enough measures will receive zero points for each measure NOT reported, unless they could not report these measures due to insufficient measures being available.

CMS will break down Quality scoring into ten categories, or "deciles," reflecting one to ten points. The deciles will be based upon stratified levels of national performance within that baseline period. The performance of each eligible clinician will be compared to the performance levels in the published deciles. Eligible clinicians will receive points based upon the decile range reflecting their level of performance. Those with performance in the top decile will receive the maximum 10 points.

All reported measures receive at least one point. Partial points are also distributed within each decile.

Bonus Score

Bonus points are available to individual clinicians and groups reporting via claims, registry, QCDR, or EHR. These may be accrued as follows:

Up to 10% for submitting high priority measures: Organizations that include high priority measures in the measures they choose to submit can receive a bonus of one to two points per measure totaling up to 10 percent of the total denominator of the Quality score (e.g. 10% of 60 = six max bonus points).

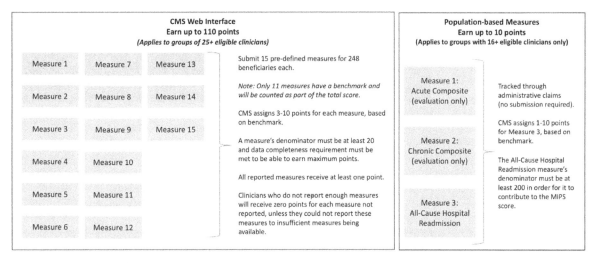

FIGURE 3-6. Scoring the Quality Category through Web Interface reporting

Up to 10% for end-to-end electronic reporting (Table 3-9): CMS is using the QPP to drive electronic reporting forward. Organizations that use end-to-end electronic reporting, which allows participants to report seamlessly from EHR to Registry without any additional human intervention, can achieve a bonus of one point for each measure totaling up to 10 percent of the possible performance points in the Quality category. Note that this bonus cap is a separate bonus cap from the high priority measures.

TABLE 3-9. End-to-End Electronic Reporting Scenarios

End-to-End Electronic Reporting Scenarios		
MIPS-eligible Clinician	Actions Taken	Then Meets End-to-End Reporting Bonus
Uses health IT certified to §170.314 or §170.315(c)(1-3)—that is, the MIPS-eligible clinician's system is certified capable of capturing, calculating, and reporting MIPS eCQMs	MIPS-eligible clinician uses their e-measure—certified health IT to submit MIPS eCQM to CMS via EHR data submission mechanism (described at 42 CFR 414.1325)	Yes
Uses health IT certified to § 170.314 or §170.315(c)(1) to capture data and export MIPS eCQM data electronically to a third-party intermediary.	The third-party intermediary is certified to be in conformance with §170.415 (c)(2-3) (import data/ calculate, report results) for each measure; and calculates and submits MIPS eCQMs.	Yes

(continued on next page)

TABLE 3-9. End-to-End Electronic Reporting Scenarios (continued)

End-to-End Electronic Reporting Scenarios		
MIPS-eligible Clinician	Actions Taken	Then Meets End-to-End Reporting Bonus
Uses health IT certified to §170.314 or §170.315(c)(1) to capture data and export a MIPS eCQM electronically to a QCDR.	QCDR uses automated, verifiable software to process data, calculate, and electronically report to a MIPS eCQM to CMS consistent with CMS-vetted protocols.	Yes
Uses certified health IT, including but not necessarily limited to that needed to satisfy the definition of CEHRT at §414.1305, to capture demographic and clinical data and transmit it to a QCDR using appropriate Clinical Document Architecture standard (such as QRDA or C-CDA)	QCDR uses automated, verifiable software to process data, calculate, and electronically report to MIPS approved non-MIPS measures consistent with CMS-vetted protocols.	Yes
Uses certified health IT, including but not necessarily limited to that needed to satisfy the definition of CEHRT at §414.1305, to capture demographic and clinical data. Makes data available to a third-party intermediary via secure application programming interface (API).	The third-party intermediary uses automated, verifiable software to process data, calculate, and electronically report to MIPS approved non-MIPS measures consistent with CMS-vetted protocols.	Yes
Uses certified health IT, including but not necessarily limited to that needed to satisfy the definition of CEHRT at §414.1305, to capture demographic and clinical data and transmit it to the third-party intermediary using appropriate standard or method (QRDA, C-CDA, API).	The eligible clinician or group, or a third-party intermediary uses automated, verifiable software to process data, calculate, and report MIPS-approved measures through manual entry, or manual manipulation of an uploaded file, into a CMS web portal.	No; manual entry interrupted data flow and electronic calculation is not verified.
Uses certified health IT to support patient care and capture data but abstracts it manually into a web portal or abstraction-input app.	The third-party intermediary uses automated, verifiable software to process data, calculate, and report measure.	No; manual abstraction interrupts data flow.

Note that the bonus points are not counted in the Quality score denominator, so it is possible to get a Quality score of greater than 100 percent, in which case the Quality score is reduced back down to 100 percent.

Clinicians can earn bonus points for submitting an additional high-priority measure, which results in:

- **Two bonus points** for each additional outcome and patient experience measure; and
- **One bonus point** for each additional high-priority measure.

Using CEHRT to submit measures to registries or CMS results in:
- **One bonus point** per measure that is submitted electronically end-to-end.

Improvement Scoring

New to the scoring component for 2018 and beyond is "Improvement Scoring" bonus points for the Quality and the Cost categories (only). As the name suggests, the bonus points available in 2018 will be for demonstrating improvement upon 2017 performance. With 2017 as the first program year for MIPS, 2018 will be the first year where these improvement bonus points will be available.

The bonus for improvement will be applied at the overall category score level. There is no measure level component available for these bonus points. By using the overall category score, CMS is allowing flexibility to providers to select any measures and/or submission methods in 2018 irrespective of what they select in 2017.

The improvement determination will be based on the "Quality Performance Category Achievement Score." This score has been defined as the Quality category score WITHOUT INCLUDING any bonus points. Also, the improvement bonus points earned in 2018 will not be included for calculating this Achievement Score in future years.

The score for 2018 would be compared to the 2017 score submitted under the same identifier defined as TIN/NPI for individual or TIN for group/APM entity. CMS has also provided guidelines if the submission identifier for an individual or a group changes in 2018 (e.g. provider leaves a group or decides to submit as an individual).

There must be a quality category performance achievement score (greater than or equal to three) for 2017 and 2018 to be eligible to receive these improvement scoring bonus points.

If the reported quality score in 2017 was less than 30 percent of the maximum possible quality score, CMS will compare to an assumed 2017 performance score of 30 percent. For most providers, the maximum quality points in 2017 were 60 points. If a clinician has fewer than 18 points (30 percent) in 2017, her 2018 score would be compared to an assumed 18 points in 2017. If you were eligible for re-admission measure in 2017, the comparison score for 2017 would be 21 (30 percent of 70). The 30 percent floor was added to ensure that a participant who used the Test Pace option in 2017 does not receive undue benefit for a low score in 2017.

A full year's participation in the Quality category is required in 2018 to be eligible for the improvement score bonus. This includes submission of all required measures and meeting data completeness criteria (Figure 3-7). The bonus points are calculated based on the following formula:

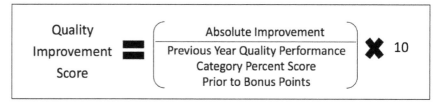

FIGURE 3-7. Quality Improvement Score

The maximum scoring improvement bonus allowed is 10 points.

There is no penalty if your Quality category performance in 2018 decreases as compared to 2017.

Calculation of Final Quality Performance Score

The improvement score bonus would be added to the quality performance category score after calculating the score based on measures, scores, and measure-based bonus points (Figure 3-8). The final Quality performance category percent score would be calculated by the following formula:

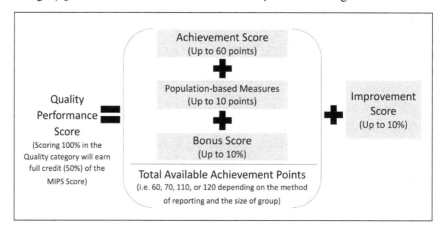

FIGURE 3-8. Calculating the Final Quality Performance Score

Remember, the Total Available Achievement Points in the denominator could be 60, 70, 110, or 120, depending on the method of reporting and size of the group.

The total category score after adding the improvement percent score cannot exceed 100 percent. Similar to 2017, this score, combined with the quality weightage, would determine the final Quality Category Score in the Composite Performance Score.

A 10 percent bonus can truly go a long way to achieving a perfect MIPS score of 100 in 2018.

Scoring Example (Table 3-10)

TABLE 3-10. Example Quality Scorecard for an Individual Clinician

Account #		Summary	Cap	Jan
Account #		Points Earned	60	22
Practice Name		High Priority Bonus Points	6	3
Example Practice Name		Bonus for add'l HP Measures	3	1
EC Name		Total HP Bonus Points	6	4
Eligible Clinician Name		CEHRT	6	6
NPI		**Total Quality Score**	**60**	**32**
#		**Quality Performance Rate**	**100**	**53**

#	HP	Description		Jan
47	Y	Advance Care Plan	Den	649
			%	0.0
110	N	Influenza Immunization	Den	157
			%	28.0
111	N	Pneumonia Immunization	Den	294
			%	32.0
128	N	BMI and Follow Up	Den	
			%	
130	Y	Documentation of Meds	Den	
			%	
137	Y	Melanoma Recall System	Den	765
			%	67.0
138	Y	Melanoma Coordination of Care	Den	806
			%	40.0
224	Y	Melanoma Overutilization of Imaging Studies	Den	509
			%	45.0
226	N	Tobacco Screening and Cessation	Den	29
			%	59.0
238	Y	High Risk Meds in the Elderly	Den	
			%	
265	Y	Biopsy Follow Up	Den	
			%	
337	N	TB Screening for Psoriasis Patients on a Biologic	Den	
			%	

When Clinicians Don't Have Enough Measures to Report

For MIPS-eligible clinicians who choose to fully participate in the MIPS program to be eligible for incentive payments, CMS states that the clinician or group must report at least six measures including at least one outcome measure if available, for a minimum of a continuous 90-day performance period. If fewer than six measures apply, then the MIPS-eligible clinician or group will only be required to report on each applicable measure.

Generally, CMS defines "applicable" to mean measures relevant to a particular MIPS-eligible clinician's services or care rendered. The MIPS-eligible clinician should be able to review a measure's specifications to see if her services fall into the denominator of the measure.

Alternatively, for a minimum of a continuous 90-day period, the MIPS-eligible clinician or group can report one specialty-specific measure set, or the measure set defined at the subspecialty level, if applicable. If the measure set contains fewer than six measures, MIPS-eligible clinicians will be required to report all available measures within the set. If the measure set contains six or more measures, MIPS-eligible clinicians can choose six or more measures to report within the set. Regardless of the number of measures that are contained in the measure set, MIPS-eligible clinicians reporting on a measure set will be required to report at least one outcome measure or, if no outcome measures are available in the measure set, report another high priority measure (appropriate use, patient safety, efficiency, patient experience, and care coordination measures) within the measure set in lieu of an outcome measure.

CMS does not believe that it is appropriate to exempt specialties from the quality performance category, even if they have fewer than six standard measures or topped out measures. Rather, these specialties are still able to report on quality measures, although for fewer measures.

CMS plans to employ multiple methods of "measure validation" to ensure that ECs are submitting the measures appropriate for them, especially when they are unable to reach the required six measures. (This process was known as the Measures Applicability Validation or "MAV" process within the PQRS program.) The MIPS measure validation process will vary according to the reporting method.

Claims or Qualified Registries: When submitting fewer than six measures through the claims or qualified data registry mechanism, CMS will utilize "cluster algorithms" from the previous PQRS MAV process to identify which measures an MIPS-eligible clinician is able to report.

Certified EHRs: CMS acknowledges that some MIPS-eligible clinicians may not have six relevant measures available within their certified EHR system. However, CMS states that if there are not six EHR measures that clinicians can submit, they should select a different reporting mechanism. ECs are also advised to work with their EHR vendors to incorporate sufficient quality measures.

QCDRs: There will not be a separate qualified clinical data registry measure validation process when quality data is submitted for QCDR participants. CMS is now requiring each QCDR to apply or reapply annually to receive QCDR status for that year, and CMS will review and approve the QCDR's measures at that time. A QCDR will not qualify for QCDR status for that year if its participants are not able to successfully report the minimum required number of measures.

Given the number of choices for submitting quality data, CMS anticipates MIPS-eligible clinicians will find a submission mechanism that meets the MIPS submission requirements. CMS strongly encourages MIPS-eligible clinicians to select the submission mechanism that has six available and appropriate measures for to their specialty and practice type.

The measure validation process exists to help individual eligible clinicians and group practices appropriately avoid the payment adjustments if they practice in specialties that have a limited number of measures for which they can report. However, MAV is an analytically complex process and while it may benefit some individual eligible professionals and group practices, it may also validate that other individual eligible professionals and group practices should be reporting more measures than they currently report.

The objective of registry-based MAV is for CMS to validate that there were no other measures applicable to the individual eligible professional's practice. This is done by reviewing the reported measures, which are inherently linked to CMS-defined measure "clusters," or groups of related measures that CMS may deem applicable to a practice.

Cluster: Measures related to a particular clinical topic or individual eligible professional service that is applicable to a specific, individual eligible professionals or group practice.

The clinical relation test will be applied to those who are subject to the validation process of satisfactorily reported measures.

The clinical relation test is based on two factors:

1. How the measure(s) satisfactorily reported currently apply within the individual eligible clinicians and group practices; and
2. The concept that if one measure in a cluster of measures related to a particular clinical topic or eligible professional service is applicable to an individual eligible professional or a group practice, then other clinically related measures within the clinical cluster **may** also be applicable. Clinical clusters within MAV are measures that are clinically related based by patient type, procedure, or possible clinical action.

Cluster: Measures related to a particular clinical topic or individual eligible professional service that is applicable to a specific, individual eligible professionals or group practice.

Beginning in 2018, individual eligible professionals and group practices who submit quality data for fewer than six quality measures will be issued a determination that decides if additional measures with additional domains may also apply to the individual eligible clinician or group practice based on their clinical cluster.

Publicly Reported Quality Measures

One of the main reasons we care so much about reporting quality measures is that much of what clinicians report to CMS will be made available to the public. In this section, we move beyond the financial impacts of quality reporting and take a look at its reputational impacts. Let's examine which quality measures are reported.

If a group practice or individual health care professional reports any of the measures designated as "available for public reporting" in the Physician Fee Schedule rule, then the measure may be included on the Physician Compare website. Only those measures deemed statistically comparable, valid, and reliable while meeting public reporting standards, including the minimum 20-patient threshold, will be considered for inclusion on the website. If the minimum threshold is not met for a particular measure, or the measure is otherwise deemed unsuitable for public reporting, the group or individual's performance rate on that measure will not be publicly reported.

Each measure title is on its own expand/collapse bar with an associated graphical representation of the percent in a series of five stars and the actual percent listed to the right. All the measures will be collapsed when a user first sees the page. A user can then expand each measure to view additional information (Figure 3-9).

▼ Controlling blood pressure in patients with diabetes.  90%

More stars are better because it means that more patients with diabetes had a controlled blood pressure measured in this group practice.

Most people with diabetes have other conditions such as high blood pressure. High blood pressure can cause heart disease and stroke. It is important to control high blood pressure to avoid additional health problems.

To give this group practice a score, Medicare looked at the percentage of this group practice's patients with diabetes whose most recent blood pressure was at a healthy level (less than 140 over 90).

FIGURE 3-9. Physician Compare Star Rating Detail

At this time, the stars are simply graphical representations of the percent. Each star represents 20 percent and so 100 percent is 5 stars, 80 percent is 4 stars, etc.

These performance scores are based on information this clinician reported to Medicare using a set of specific criteria and guidelines developed to show whether this doctor provided patients the best-recommended care. Performance scores are included on Physician Compare to help you make informed decisions about your health care and to encourage all clinicians to improve the care they provide. It's important to understand that not all clinicians report the same information to Medicare, and the types of care available to report on differ depending on the types of services they provide to patients. Reporting more or less information is not a reflection of this clinician's quality. Also, the performance scores do not form a complete picture of the types of services this clinician provides. This is just a snapshot of some of the care this clinician provided to people with Medicare in 2015.

The data is updated often, as frequently as once a month, and once we complete the first MIPS reporting year, this is the website that will publish your MIPS scores, including category level details.

If you have not done so already, I invite you to visit the *medicare.gov/ physiciancompare* website to review your practice and clinician profiles. You can see if there are any errors or mistakes on your page and really start to wrap your head around what quality data is reported now and will be reported in the future.

Keys to Success

- Focus on taking good care of patients with chronic conditions.
- Treat acute conditions early to avoid hospitalizations.
- Choose relevant measures and focus on performance rates.
- Be familiar with your Quality and Resource Use Report (QRUR) as far back as possible. (As yourself: Where am I in respect to the benchmarks for both CMS-calculated measures and submitted quality measures?)
- Provide complete follow-ups with patients post-hospitalization to keep the All-Cause Hospital Readmissions score low.
- Be patient-centered and have hassle-free accessibility.
- Aim to get those bonus points!

Resources

- https://qpp.cms.gov/mips/quality-measures
- QPP Resource Library Documents: https://www.cms.gov/Medicare/ Quality-Payment-Program/Resource-Library/2018-Resources.html
  — 2018 Quality Measure Specifications
  — 2018 MIPS Quality Performance Category Fact Sheet
  — 2018 Quality Benchmarks
  — 2018 Qualified Registries
  — 2018 CMS-Approved Qualified Clinical Data Registries (QCDRs)

— CAHPS for MIPS Fact Sheet: https://www.cms.gov/Medicare/Quality-Payment-Program/Resource-Library/CAHPS-for-MIPS-Fact-Sheet.pdf
— CMS Web Interface Fact Sheet: https://www.cms.gov/Medicare/Quality-Payment-Program/Resource-Library/CMS-Web-Interface-Fact-Sheet-2.pdf
— CMS Web Interface Excel Instructions: https://www.cms.gov/Medicare/Quality-Payment-Program/Resource-Library/CMS-Web-Interface-Excel-Template-User-Guide-2017.pdf
— Registration Instructions for CAHPS for MIPS and CMS Web Interface: https://qpp.cms.gov/mips/individual-or-group-participation/about-group-registration
— MAV information: https://www.cms.gov/Medicare/Quality-Initiatives-Patient-Assessment-Instruments/PQRS/Downloads/2016_PQRS_MAV_ProcessforRegistryBasedReporting_030716.pdf

Lessons Learned from the Field

Lesson 1: Take advantage of Intake Forms!

In an effort to reduce the burden of data collection, consider the many quality measures where you can get credit for simply asking the patient a question, and documenting the response. One way to tackle this is to update your intake form with the relevant questions and have the patient do the heavy lifting. Examples include:

• Have you had your flu shot?
• Have you ever had a pneumonia vaccination?
• Are you a current smoker?
• Do you consume alcohol? If so, how much?
• Do you have advance directives on file?

In these examples, it is not necessary for the clinician to actually administer the immunization or vaccination. Rather, documenting the patient's results and recommending that they get the needed treatments counts as meeting the measure's requirements.

Lesson 2: Know your "inverse" measures.

For some quality measures, a lower performance rate indicates better clinical care or control and therefore produces a higher score. These are called "Inverse" measures.

One commonly used inverse measure is "Use of High-Risk Medication in the Elderly," which measures how many patients aged 65 and older are prescribed medications that are listed as high-risk because they may alter the patient's psychological state.

Another commonly used inverse measure is "Diabetes A1c Poor Control," which tracks patients between ages 18 to75 who have a diagnosis of diabetes and had a hemoglobin A1c greater than nine percent. The lower the patient's result, the better the patient's diabetes is being managed. If the A1c measurement is higher than nine percent, the patient may have a higher chance of complications while managing her diabetes.

As you can imagine, the closer to zero the clinician's performance rate for both of these measures, the better.

Lesson 3: If interfacing your EHR with a registry, give it time.

Anytime you try to get two technology systems to share information, there are opportunities for errors. When information is pushed, pulled, or sometimes both, from one system to another, each field that contains data to be transported must be cross-walked and mapped accurately, so that data is taken from the right place in one application and also lands in the correct place within the other.

Know that this process takes time. There was one particular data mapping issue between an EHR and a registry that delayed heaps of practices for months, which meant that the clinicians couldn't get an accurate view of their data until the two systems worked together to correct the mapping errors.

If you are considering interfacing your EHR with a registry, factor in enough time in your implementation schedule to account for this type of delay.

Lesson 4: For claims-based reporters, there is no easy way to document a missed opportunity.

Claims-based reporting may be one of the most straightforward methods to report quality measure data, but the significance of having a solid workflow in place to consistently capture the accurate codes on each claim cannot be understated.

If an opportunity is missed, the opportunity to increase your numerator is gone, while your denominator will continue to grow, resulting in a lower performance rate.

ADVANCING CARE INFORMATION (ACI)

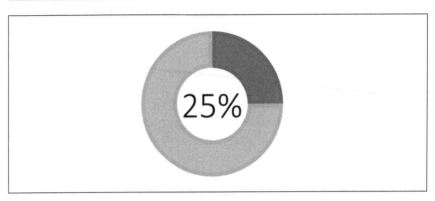

FIGURE 3-10. 2018 Advancing Care Information Weight

The Advancing Care Information (ACI) draws directly from the Medicare EHR Incentive Program (i.e. Meaningful Use), as many of its features are simply repackaged and repurposed Meaningful Use requirements. As a reminder, the primary goal of the Medicare EHR Incentive Program was to encourage and promote the adoption and use of electronic health records (EHR) among Medicare and Medicaid healthcare providers to help drive the industry as a whole toward a more standardized use of EHRs (Figure 3-10).

CMS's approach to reporting the ACI category is much more customizable and flexible than the previous iteration, allowing clinicians, for the most part, to choose which objectives and measures best fit their practice. This tactic offers multiple paths for success.

Health information exchange and patient engagement are among the more challenging objectives, but are both essential to leveraging EHR technology to improve care coordination. These areas represent the greatest potential for improvement and for significant impact on healthcare delivery.

Considering this, their new framework moves away from the concept of requiring a single threshold for a measure, and instead encourages continuous improvement, recognizing the challenges that clinicians face with adopting and implementing EHR technology into their practices. CMS has learned that updating software, training staff, and changing practice workflows to accommodate new technology takes time, and that clinicians need time and flexibility to focus on the health IT activities that are most relevant to their patient population.

The new ACI framework focuses on these high-impact objectives, which are essential to leveraging EHR technology to improve care:

- Patient Electronic Access
- Coordination of Care Through Patient Engagement
- Health Information Exchange

Their approach also de-emphasizes objectives in which clinicians have historically achieved high performance in years past. This mainly includes the computerized provider order entry (CPOE) and clinical decision support rules (CDS) objectives, which can be easily achieved by configuring the EHR and modifying workflows.

In future years, CMS may adopt more stringent measures and establish benchmarks for the ACI category measures, similar to their approach for Quality. They may even introduce improvement scoring in the ACI category as a comparison for the subsequent year's category score. These types of approaches would drive continuous improvement forward over time. Eventually, CMS wants to be able to tie patient health outcomes with the use of health IT. However, the technology and measurement for this type of program is not currently available.

EHR Certification Edition

In speaking to the mass adoption of EHRs that has taken place in the past several years, the fact of the matter is that some EHR vendors have been able to keep up with the government's suggested development pace, while other vendors have lagged. This development gap often shows up in the form of limitations to what clinicians can accomplish within their EHR.

To address this problem, CMS has allowed for the use of two separate editions of EHR technology to be used in order to meet the ACI category requirements for both the 2017 and 2018 performance years. This is meant to offer the EHR vendors time to close their development gaps, while providing flexibility for clinicians, based on the edition to which their EHR is certified.

Clinicians will find that their EHR is certified to either the 2014 Edition standard or the 2015 Edition standard.

The 2014 Edition standard was originally adopted in 2012 to meet the technical requirements specified as part of the EHR Incentive Program. The 2015 Edition stemmed from the collection of criteria created for previous versions to facilitate greater interoperability among systems for clinical purposes as well as to better enable the exchange of health information.

The 2014 Edition was the standard used to attest to Meaningful Use in 2015 and 2016. For clinicians who are still using a 2014 Edition certified EHR, reporting ACI will look and feel very similar to the Meaningful Use reporting they had done in the past. They will submit on the same objectives that were included in their EHR's "Modified Stage 2" report.

Much of the new functionality in 2015 Edition EHR certification lends itself to offering patients more access to their health information, allowing them to share it more easily through application programming interfaces

CMIS is offering bonuses to clinicians who upgrade and only use 2015 Edition EHR technology in 2018.

(APIs), and to engage more actively in their own care. As more providers across the healthcare continuum upgrade to this technical standard, they are forming an essential foundation for interoperability and are helping to ensure that key data is consistently available to the right person, at the right place, at the right time.

The 2015 Edition is also set up to safeguard highly sensitive health information related to certain conditions that receive special protection under the law. It allows for additional and more precise patient information fields that will help to match patient records—and even information from their implantable devices—more accurately and precisely.

This Edition addresses health disparities by supporting the capture of patient health information with more granularity that will be able to help clinicians identify opportunities for care improvement for the patient populations that they serve. This includes a more granular capture of race and ethnicity data, social, psychological, and behavioral health data, as well as data on sexual orientation/gender identity, when a patient chooses to self-identify this demographic information. It contains functionality to support the standardized exchange of sensitive health information, filtering of clinical quality measure data to identify health disparities, and the capture of health information directly from patients.

Throughout the 2018 program year, CMS anticipates that all certified EHR technologies will be updated to meet the 2015 Edition standards, so that by the time the 2019 program year begins, all clinicians will have upgraded to the newer version.

Below, we will detail the requirements for both EHR options. You will notice that they share many similarities, but also some very important and distinct differences as well.

In both options, CMS outlines the Base, Performance, and Bonus scores that will make up the full category score. We will review all three score types for each option.

CMIS is offering bonuses to clinicians who upgrade and only use 2015 Edition EHR technology in 2018.

Option 1—2014 Edition EHR

A MIPS-eligible clinician who has an EHR certified to the 2014 Edition is capable of reporting:
- Four Base Objectives
  — Protect Patient Health Information
  — e-Prescribing
  — Provide Patient Access
  — Health Information Exchange (HIE): Send Summary of Care

TABLE 3-11. 2014 Edition certified EHR technology Base Point Requirements

		2014 Edition CEHRT Base Points	
		(A requirement to meet in order to earn *any* points in the ACI performance category in the 2018 program year)	
Objective	**Measure**	**Description**	**Reporting Requirement**
Protect Patient Health Information	Security Risk Analysis	Conduct or review a security risk analysis in accordance with the requirements in 45 CFR 164.308(a)(1), including addressing the security (to include encryption) of ePHI data created or maintained by CEHRT in accordance with requirements in 45 CFR164.312(a)(2)(iv) and 45 CFR 164.306(d)(3), and implement security updates as necessary and correct identified security deficiencies as part of the MIPS-eligible clinician's risk management process.	Yes/No Statement
Electronic Prescribing*	e-Prescribing	At least one permissible prescription written by the MIPS-eligible clinician is queried for a drug formulary and transmitted electronically using CEHRT.	Numerator/ Denominator
Patient Electronic Access	Provide Patient Access	At least one patient seen by the MIPS-eligible clinician during the performance period is provided timely access to view online, download, and transmit to a third party their health information subject to the MIPS-eligible clinician's discretion to withhold certain information.	Numerator/ Denominator
Health Information Exchange*	Send Summary of Care	The MIPS-eligible clinician that transitions or refers her patient to another setting of care or health care clinician (1) uses CEHRT to create a summary of care record; and (2) electronically transmits such summary to a receiving health care clinician for at least one transition of care or referral.	Numerator/ Denominator

Exclusion available.

- Seven Performance Objectives
  — Provide Patient Access
  — View, Download, Transmit
  — Patient Specific Education
  — Secure Messaging
  — HIE: Send Summary of Care
  — Medication Reconciliation
  — Immunization Registry Reporting
- Three Bonus Objectives
  — Special Registry Reporting
  — Syndromic Surveillance Reporting
  — Report Improvement Activities Using Certified EHR Technology

Let's dig a little deeper into each area, beginning with the Base points.

To earn *any* points in the ACI category, the Base objectives must be met at least one time. This means that the clinician must attest to each of these four objectives with a "Yes" statement and/or a minimum of 1/1 for the numerator/denominator where applicable (Table 3-11).

This next section includes important definitions and "additional information" that is taken directly from the ACI measures specification sheets for each of these Base objectives. Oftentimes, you'll find the answers to your questions about objectives in these documents that live in the QPP resource library.

Protect Patient Information: To meet this measure, MIPS-eligible clinicians must attest YES to conducting or reviewing a security risk analysis and implementing security updates as necessary and correcting identified security deficiencies.

e-Prescribing: A MIPS-eligible clinician should use CEHRT as the sole means of creating the prescription, and when transmitting to an external pharmacy that is independent of the MIPS-eligible clinician's organization, though such transmission must use standards adopted for EHR technology certification.

e-Prescribing Exclusion Criteria: Any MIPS-eligible clinician who writes fewer than 100 permissible prescriptions during the performance period.

Clinicians may claim this exclusion if they qualify, although they do not have to claim the exclusion and may report on the measure if they choose to do so.

Provide Patient Access: When a patient possesses all of the tools and information needed to gain access to their health information including, but not limited to, any necessary instructions, user identification information, or the steps required to access their information if they have previously elected to "opt out" of electronic access.

To meet this measure, the following information must be made available to patients electronically:

- Patient name
- Provider's name and office contact information
- Current and past problem list
- Procedures
- Laboratory test results
- Current medication list and medication history
- Current medication allergy list and medication allergy history
- Vital signs (height, weight, blood pressure, BMI, growth charts)
- Smoking status
- Demographic information (preferred language, sex, race, ethnicity, date of birth)

- Care plan field(s), including goals and instructions
- Any known care team members including the primary care provider (PCP) of record

If a patient elects to "opt out" of participation, the MIPS-eligible clinician may count that patient in the numerator if the patient is provided all of the necessary information to subsequently access her information, obtain access through a patient-authorized representative, or otherwise opt back in without further follow up action required by the clinician.

Health Information Exchange:

Transition of Care—The movement of a patient from one setting of care (hospital, ambulatory primary care practice, ambulatory, specialty care practice, long-term care, home health, rehabilitation facility) to another. At a minimum, this includes all transitions of care and referrals that are ordered by the MIPS-eligible clinician.

Summary of Care Record—All summary of care documents used to meet this measure must include the following information if the MIPS-eligible clinician knows it:

- Patient name
- Referring or transitioning healthcare provider's name and office contact information (MIPS-eligible clinician only)
- Procedures
- Encounter diagnosis
- Immunizations
- Laboratory test results
- Vital signs (height, weight, blood pressure, BMI)
- Smoking status
- Functional status, including activities of daily living, cognitive, and disability status
- Demographic information (preferred language, sex, race, ethnicity, date of birth)
- Care plan field, including goals and instructions
- Care team, including the primary care provider of record and any additional known care team members beyond the referring or transitioning provider and the receiving provider
- Reason for referral (MIPS-eligible clinician only)
- Current problem list (Providers may also include historical problems at their discretion)*
- Current medication list*
- Current medication allergy list*

*Note: A MIPS-eligible clinician must verify that the fields for the current problem list, current medication list, and current medication allergy list are not blank and include the most recent information known by the MIPS-eligible clinician at the time of generating the summary of care document or include a notation of no current problem, medication and/or medication allergies.

Current problem lists—At a minimum, a list of current and active diagnoses.

Active/current medication list—A list of medications that a given patient is currently taking.

Active/current medication allergy list—A list of medications to which a given patient has known allergies.

Allergy—An exaggerated immune response or reaction to substances that are generally not harmful.

Care Plan—The structure used to define the management actions for the various conditions, problems, or issues. A care plan must include, at a minimum, the following components: problem (the focus of the care plan), goal (the target outcome), and any instructions that the MIPS-eligible clinician has given to the patient. A goal is a defined target or measure to be achieved in the process of patient care (an expected outcome).

HIE Exclusion Criteria: Any MIPS-eligible clinician who transfers a patient to another setting or refers a patient fewer than 100 times during the performance period can exclude this objective.

Clinicians may claim this exclusion if they qualify, although they do not have to claim it and may report on the measure if they choose to do so.

By achieving these four Base objectives, you can earn half of the points available for this category: 50 out of 100, which translates to 12.5 of the 25 percent contribution to the final MIPS score.

If you are solely interested in avoiding a penalty, completing these four tasks would get you pretty close to that goal.

To build on that score, you would need to show that you have achieved performance in any of the seven objectives included in the Performance Points outlined in Table 3-12. Reporting on any of these objectives is not mandatory. Instead, you can focus on the ones that are meaningful to you or relatively easy to achieve. Offering this level of flexibility allows you to reach the full category score through a path of your own choosing.

TABLE 3-12. 2014 Edition Certified EHR Technology Performance Point Requirements

2014 Edition CEHRT Performance Points				
Objective	Measure	Description	Performance Score	Reporting Requirement
Patient Electronic Access	Provide Patient Access	At least one patient seen by the MIPS-eligible clinician during the performance period is provided timely access to view online, download, and transmit to a third party their health information subject to the MIPS-eligible clinician's discretion to withhold certain information.	Up to 20 Points	Numerator/ Denominator
Patient Electronic Access	View, Download, or Transmit (VDT)	At least one patient seen by the MIPS-eligible clinician during the performance period (or patient-authorized representative) views, downloads or transmits their health information to a third party during the performance period.	Up to 10 Points	Numerator/ Denominator
Patient Specific Education	Patient Specific Education	The MIPS-eligible clinician must use clinically relevant information from CEHRT to identify patient-specific educational resources and provide access to those materials to at least one unique patient seen by the MIPS-eligible clinician.	Up to 10 Points	Numerator/ Denominator
Secure Messaging	Secure Messaging	For at least one patient seen by the MIPS-eligible clinician during the performance period, a secure message was sent using the electronic messaging function of CEHRT to the patient (or the patient- authorized representative), or in response to a secure message sent by the patient (or the patient authorized representative), during the performance period.	Up to 10 Points	Numerator/ Denominator
Health Information Exchange	Send Summary of Care	The MIPS-eligible clinician that transitions or refers their patient to another setting of care or health care clinician (1) uses CEHRT to create a summary of care record; and (2) electronically transmits such summary to a receiving health care clinician for at least one transition of care or referral.	Up to 20 Points	Numerator/ Denominator
Medication Reconciliation	Medication Reconciliation	The MIPS-eligible clinician performs medication reconciliation for at least one transition of care in which the patient is transitioned into the care of the MIPS-eligible clinician.	Up to 10 Points	Numerator/ Denominator
Public Health Reporting	Immunization Registry	The MIPS-eligible clinician is in active engagement with a public health agency to submit immunization data.	0 or 10 Points	Numerator/ Denominator

There are a total of 90 points available in the Performance section, which if all available points we've covered so far were earned, would give a clinician 140 category points. It's important to know that CMS caps the aggregate score at 100.

One thing to notice is that there are two objectives here that are worth up to 20 points whereas the rest are only worth up to 10. These two are:

- Providing patients access to their health data; and
- Health Information Exchange, sending a summary of care.

These objectives align very well with the overarching themes of the Quality Payment Program and CMS is weighing them more heavily than the others in this subset to provide you with the opportunity to still earn up to 90 points in the Performance section.

This next section includes important definitions and "additional information" that is taken directly from the ACI measures specification sheets for each of these Performance objectives.

Provide Patient Access: Keen eyes will notice that this objective was also included in the Base points. In the Base section, CMS is only interested in whether this objective was met *one time*. In the Performance Score section, CMS takes into account the performance rate for the entire reporting period.

For this objective, you are tasked with giving patients electronic access to their health information through a patient portal, patient health record, or similar mechanism/feature.

Provide Access—When a patient possesses all of the tools and information needed to gain access to her health information, including, but not limited to any necessary instructions, user identification information, or the steps required to access her information if she has previously elected to "opt out" of electronic access.

View, Download, and Transmit (VDT): Once patients have been provided electronic access to their health information, CMS wants to know how many patients actually logged in to view it. The VDT objective measures how often patients went online to view, download, or transmit their personal information to another healthcare provider.

View—The patient (or authorized representative) accessing their health information online.

Download—The movement of information from online to physical electronic media.

Transmission—This may be any means of electronic transmission according to any transport standard(s) (e.g., SMTP, FTP, REST, SOAP, etc.). However, the relocation of physical electronic media (e.g., USB or CD) does not qualify as transmission.

Diagnostic Test Results—All data needed to diagnose and treat disease. Examples include, but are not limited to blood tests, microbiology, urinalysis, pathology tests, radiology, cardiac imaging, nuclear medicine tests, and pulmonary function tests.

The patient must be able to access this information on demand, such as through a patient portal via personal health record (PHR), or by other online electronic means.

Patient-Specific Education:

Patient-Specific Education Resources Identified by CEHRT—Resources or a topic area of resources identified through logic built into certified EHR technology, which evaluate information about the patient and suggest education resources that would be of value to the patient.

The MIPS-eligible clinician must use elements within CEHRT to identify educational resources specific to patients' needs. CEHRT is certified to use the patient's problem list, medication list, or laboratory test results to identify the patient-specific educational resources. The MIPS-eligible clinician may use these or additional elements within CEHRT to identify educational resources specific to patients' needs. The MIPS-eligible clinician can then provide these educational resources to patients in a useful, viewer-friendly format (such as electronic copy, printed copy, electronic link to source materials, through a patient portal, or PHR).

The education resources or materials do not need to be stored within or generated electronically by the CEHRT.

There is no universal "transitive effect" policy in place for this measure. It may vary based on the resources and materials provided and the timing of that provision. If an action is clearly attributable to a single clinician, it may only count in the numerator for that clinician. However, if the action is not attributable to a single MIPS-eligible clinician, it may be counted in the numerator for all MIPS-eligible clinicians sharing the CEHRT who have contributed information to the patient's record and who have the patient in their denominator for the MIPS performance period.

Secure Messaging:

Secure Message—Any electronic communication between a MIPS-eligible clinician and patient that ensures only those parties can access the communication. This electronic message could be communicated via email or the electronic messaging function of a personal health record (PHR), an online patient portal, or any other electronic means.

Fully Enabled—The function is fully installed, any security measures are fully enabled, and the function is readily available for patient use.

HIE: Send Summary of Care: See the description from the 2014 Edition Base points section. The information is the same.

Medication Reconciliation:

Medication Reconciliation—The process of identifying the most accurate list of all medications that the patient is taking—including name, dosage, frequency, and route—by comparing the medical record to an external list of medications obtained from a patient, hospital, or other healthcare provider.

Transition of Care—The movement of a patient from one setting of care (hospital, ambulatory primary care practice, ambulatory, specialty care practice, long-term care, home health, rehabilitation facility) to another. At a minimum, this includes all transitions of care and referrals that are ordered by the MIPS-eligible clinician.

Referral—Cases where one MIPS-eligible clinician refers a patient to another, but the referring clinician maintains his or her care of the patient as well.

Denominator for Transitions of Care and Referrals—The denominator includes transitions of care and referrals.

In the case of reconciliation following transition of care, the receiving MIPS-eligible clinician should conduct the medication reconciliation.

The electronic exchange of information is not a requirement for medication reconciliation and this measure does not dictate what information must be included in medication reconciliation. The provider and patient determine information appropriate for inclusion in the process of medication reconciliation.

Public Health Reporting, Immunization Registry:

Active engagement—the MIPS-eligible clinician is in the process of moving towards sending "production data" to a public health agency (PHA) or clinical data registry (CDR), or is sending production data to a PHA or CDR.

Active engagement may be demonstrated in one of the following ways:

Option 1—Completed Registration to Submit Data: The MIPS-eligible clinician registered to submit data with the PHA or, where applicable, the CDR to which the information is being submitted; registration was completed within 60 days after the start of the MIPS performance period; and the MIPS-eligible clinician is awaiting an invitation from

TABLE 3-13. 2014 Edition certified EHR technology Bonus Point Requirements

2014 Edition CEHRT Bonus Points				
Objective	Measure	Description	Performance Score	Reporting Requirement
Public Health Reporting	Syndromic Surveillance Reporting	The MIPS-eligible clinician is in active engagement with a public health agency to submit syndromic surveillance data.	Up to 10 Points	Yes/No Statement
Public Health Reporting	Specialized Registry Reporting	The MIPS-eligible clinician is in active engagement to submit data to a specialized registry.	Up to 10 Points	Yes/No Statement
Report Improvement Activities using CEHRT			10 Points	Yes/No Statement

the PHA or CDR to begin testing and validation. This option allows MIPS-eligible clinicians to meet the measure when the PHA or the CDR has limited resources to initiate the testing and validation process. MIPS-eligible clinicians who have registered in previous years do not need to submit an additional registration to meet this requirement for each MIPS performance period.

Option 2—Testing and Validation: The MIPS-eligible clinician is in the process of testing and validation of the electronic submission of data. MIPS-eligible clinicians must respond to requests from the PHA or, where applicable, the CDR within 30 days; failure to respond twice within a MIPS performance period would result in that MIPS-eligible clinician not meeting the measure.

Option 3—Production: The MIPS-eligible clinician has completed testing and validation of the electronic submission and is electronically submitting production data to the PHA or CDR.

MIPS-eligible clinicians who have previously registered, tested, or begun ongoing submission of data to the registry are not required to "restart" the process by beginning at active engagement Option 1. The MIPS-eligible clinician may simply attest to the active engagement option that most closely reflects their current status (Table 3-13).

Public Health Reporting, Syndromic Surveillance Registry:

These share the same definitions as the Immunization Registry.

Earning bonus points for this measure is not contingent upon the reporting of the Advancing Care Information performance score measures.

Public Health Reporting, Specialized Registry:

Same definitions as Immunization Registry.

Earning bonus points for this measure is not contingent upon the reporting of the Advancing Care Information performance score measures.

Report Improvement Activities using CEHRT:

There is a subset of Improvement Activities that award you bonus points in the ACI category, specifically, when an Improvement Activity uses Certified EHR to achieve it. When choosing your Improvement Activities, consider which of these measures will afford you a 10-point bonus in the ACI category.

Option 2—2015 Edition

A MIPS-eligible clinician who has an EHR certified to the 2015 Edition is capable of reporting:

- Five Base Score Objectives
  — Protect Patient Health Information
  — e-Prescribing
  — Provide Patient Access
  — Health Information Exchange (HIE): Send Summary of Care
  — Health Information Exchange (HIE): Request/Accept Summary of Care
- Nine Performance Score Objectives
  — Provide Patient Access
  — Patient Education
  — View, Download, Transmit
  — Secure Messaging
  — Patient Generated Health Data
  — HIE: Send Summary of Care
  — HIE: Request/Accept Summary of Care
  — Clinician Information Reconciliation
  — Immunization Registry Reporting
- Six Bonus Score Objectives
  — Syndromic Surveillance Reporting
  — Electronic Case Reporting
  — Public Health Registry Reporting
  — Clinical Data Registry Reporting
  — Report Improvement Activities using Certified EHR Technology
  — Using 2015 Edition CEHRT for the Entire Reporting Period

Let's review each area, beginning with the Base points (Table 3-14).

TABLE 3-14. 2015 Edition certified EHR technology Base Point Requirements

2015 Edition CEHRT Base Points (Required to meet in order to earn *any* points in the ACI performance category in the 2018 program year)			
Objective	Measure	Description	Reporting Requirement
Protect Patient Health Information	Security Risk Analysis	Conduct or review a security risk analysis in accordance with the requirements in 45 CFR 164.308(a)(1), including addressing the security (to include encryption) of ePHI data created or maintained by CEHRT in accordance with requirements in 45 CFR164.312(a)(2)(iv) and 45 CFR 164.306(d)(3), implement security updates as necessary, and correct identified security deficiencies as part of the MIPS-eligible clinician's risk management process.	Yes/No Statement
Electronic Prescribing*	e-Prescribing	At least one permissible prescription written by the MIPS-eligible clinician is queried for a drug formulary and transmitted electronically using CEHRT.	Numerator/ Denominator
Patient Electronic Access	Provide Patient Access	At least one patient seen by the MIPS -eligible clinician during the performance period is provided timely access to view online, download, and transmit to a third party their health information subject to the MIPS-eligible clinician's discretion to withhold certain information.	Numerator/ Denominator
Health Information Exchange*	Send Summary of Care	For at least one transition of care or referral, the MIPS-eligible clinician that transitions or refers her patient to another setting of care or health care clinician—(1) creates a summary of care record using CEHRT; and (2) electronically exchanges the summary of care record.	Numerator/ Denominator
Health Information Exchange*	Request/ Accept Summary of Care	For at least one transition of care or referral received or patient encounter in which the MIPS-eligible clinician has never before encountered the patient, the MIPS-eligible clinician receives or retrieves and incorporates into the patient's record an electronic summary of care document.	Numerator/ Denominator

* Exclusion available.

Attesting to each of these five objectives with a "Yes" statement and/or a minimum of 1/1 for the numerator/denominator, where applicable, will earn the clinician half of the points available for this category.

This next section includes important definitions and "additional information" that is taken directly from the ACI measures specification sheets for each of these Base objectives. Oftentimes, you'll find the answers to your questions about objectives in these documents that live in the QPP resource library.

Protect Patient Information: To meet this measure, MIPS-eligible clinicians must attest YES to conducting or reviewing a security risk analysis and implementing security updates as necessary while also correcting identified security deficiencies.

e-Prescribing: A MIPS-eligible clinician needs to use CEHRT as the sole means of creating the prescription, and when transmitting to an external pharmacy that is independent of the MIPS-eligible clinician's organization, the transmission must use standards adopted for EHR technology certification.

e-Prescribing Exclusion Criteria: Any MIPS-eligible clinician who writes fewer than 100 permissible prescriptions during the performance period.

Clinicians may claim this exclusion if they qualify to do so, although they do not have to claim the exclusion and may report on the measure if they so choose.

Provide Patient Access:

The Provide Patient Access measure is critical to increasing patient engagement, and to allowing patients access to their personal health data in order to improve health, provide transparency, and drive patient engagement.

Provide Patient Access: When a patient possesses all of the tools and information needed to gain access to her health information including, but not limited to, any necessary instructions, user identification information, or the steps required to access a patient's information if she has previously elected to "opt out" of electronic access.

API or Application Programming Interface—A set of programming protocols established for multiple purposes. APIs may be enabled by a health care provider or health care provider organization to provide the patient with access to his health information through a third-party application with more flexibility than is often found in many current "patient portals."

To meet this measure, the following information must be made available to patients electronically:
- Patient name
- Provider's name and office contact information
- Current and past problem list
- Procedures
- Laboratory test results
- Current medication list and medication history
- Current medication allergy list and medication allergy history
- Vital signs (height, weight, blood pressure, BMI, growth charts)
- Smoking status
- Demographic information (preferred language, sex, race, ethnicity, date of birth)

- Care plan field(s), including goals and instructions
- Any known care team members including the primary care provider (PCP) of record

The patient must be able to access this information on demand, such as through a patient portal or personal health record (PHR) or by other online electronic means.

If a patient elects to "opt out" of participation, the MIPS-eligible clinician may count that patient in the numerator if the patient is provided all of the necessary information to subsequently access her information, obtain access through a patient-authorized representative, or otherwise opt back in without further follow up action required by the clinician.

Health Information Exchange: Send a Summary of Care & Request/Accept Summary of Care

Send a Summary of Care

Transition of Care—The movement of a patient from one setting of care (e.g., hospital, ambulatory primary care practice, ambulatory, specialty care practice, long-term care, home health, or rehabilitation facility) to another. At a minimum, this includes all transitions of care and referrals that are ordered by the MIPS-eligible clinician.

Summary of Care Record—All summary of care documents used to meet this measure must include the following information if the MIPS-eligible clinician knows it:

- Patient name
- Referring or transitioning healthcare provider's name and office contact information (MIPS-eligible clinician only)
- Procedures
- Encounter diagnosis
- Immunizations
- Laboratory test results
- Vital signs (height, weight, blood pressure, BMI)
- Smoking status
- Functional status, including activities of daily living, cognitive and disability status
- Demographic information (preferred language, sex, race, ethnicity, date of birth)
- Care plan field, including goals and instructions
- Care team including the primary care provider of record and any additional known care team members beyond the referring or transitioning provider and the receiving provider

- Reason for referral (MIPS-eligible clinician only)
- Current problem list (Providers may also include historical problems at their discretion)*
- Current medication list*
- Current medication allergy list*

Note: A MIPS-eligible clinician must verify that the fields for current problem list, current medication list, and current medication allergy list are not blank and include the most recent information known by the MIPS-eligible clinician at the time of generating the summary of care document or include a notation of no current problem, medication, and/or medication allergies.

Current Problem List—At a minimum, a list of current and active diagnoses.

Active/current medication List—A list of medications that a given patient is currently taking.

Active/Current Medication Allergy list—A list of medications to which a given patient has known allergies.

Allergy—An exaggerated immune response or reaction to substances that are generally not harmful.

Care Plan—The structure used to define the management actions for the various conditions, problems, or issues. A care plan must include, at a minimum, the following components: problem (the focus of the care plan), goal (the target outcome), and any instructions that the MIPS-eligible clinician has given to the patient. A goal is a defined target or measure to be achieved in the process of patient care (an expected outcome).

For the measure, only patients whose records are maintained using certified EHR technology must be included in the denominator for transitions of care.

This exchange may occur before, during, or after the MIPS performance period. However, it must occur within the calendar year to count in the numerator.

A MIPS-eligible clinician must have confirmation of receipt or that a query of the summary of care record has occurred in order to count the action in the numerator.

In cases where the MIPS-eligible clinicians share access to an EHR, a transition or referral may still count toward the measure if the referring health care provider creates the summary of care document using CEHRT and electronically submits the summary of care document. If a MIPS-eligible clinician chooses to include such transitions to clinicians where access to the EHR is shared, they must do so universally for all patient and all transitions or referrals.

The initiating MIPS-eligible clinician must send a C–CDA document that the receiving clinician would be capable of electronically incorporating as a C–CDA on the receiving end. In other words, if a MIPS-eligible clinician sends a C–CDA and the receiving clinician converts the C–CDA into a pdf, a fax or some other format, the sending health care provider may still count the transition or referral in the numerator. If the sending MIPS-eligible clinician converts the file to a format the receiving clinician could not electronically receive and incorporate as a C–CDA, the initiating clinician may not count the transition in their numerator.

Request/Accept Summary of Care

For the purposes of defining the cases in the denominator for the measure, CMS states that the following descriptions constitute "unavailable" and, therefore, may be excluded from the denominator. The label is appropriate when an MIPS-eligible-clinician:

- Requested an electronic summary of care record to be sent and did not receive an electronic summary of care document; and
- The MIPS-eligible clinician either:
  — Queried at least one external source via HIE functionality and did not locate a summary of care for the patient, or the clinician does not have access to HIE functionality to support such a query, or
  — Confirmed that HIE functionality-supporting query for summary of care documents was not operational in the MIPS-eligible clinician's geographic region and not available within the clinician's EHR network as of the start of the MIPS performance period.

For the measure, a record cannot be considered incorporated if it is discarded without the reconciliation of clinical information or if it is stored in a manner that is not accessible for clinician use within the EHR.

HIE Exclusion Criteria: Any MIPS-eligible clinician who transfers a patient to another setting or refers a patient fewer than 100 times during the performance period can exclude this objective.

Clinicians may claim this exclusion if they qualify, although they do not have to claim the exclusion and may report on the measure if they choose to do so.

TABLE 3-15. 2015 Edition Certified EHR Technology Performance Point Requirements

2015 Edition CEHRT Performance Points				
Objective	Measure	Description	Performance Score	Reporting Requirement
Patient Electronic Access	Provide Patient Access	For at least one unique patient seen by the MIPS-eligible clinician: (1) The patient (or the patient-authorized representative) is provided timely access to view online, download, and transmit his or her health information; and (2) The MIPS-eligible clinician ensures the patient's health information is available for the patient (or patient-authorized representative) to access using any application of her choice that is configured to meet the technical specifications of the Application Programing Interface (API) in the MIPS-eligible clinician's CEHRT.	Up to 10 Points	Numerator/ Denominator
Patient Electronic Access	Patient Education	The MIPS-eligible clinician must use clinically relevant information from CEHRT to identify patient-specific educational resources and provide electronic access to those materials to at least one unique patient seen by the MIPS-eligible clinician.	Up to 10 Points	Numerator/ Denominator
Coordination of Care Through Patient Engagement	View, Download, or Transmit (VDT)	During the performance period, at least one unique patient (or patient-authorized representatives) seen by the MIPS-eligible clinician actively engages with the EHR made accessible by the MIPS-eligible clinician. A MIPS-eligible clinician may meet the measure by either—(1) view, download or transmit to a third party their health information; or (2) access their health information through the use of an API that can be used by applications chosen by the patient and configured to the API in the MIPS-eligible clinician's CEHRT; or (3) a combination of (1) and (2).	Up to 10 Points	Numerator/ Denominator
Coordination of Care Through Patient Engagement	Secure Messaging	For at least one patient seen by the MIPS-eligible clinician during the performance period, a secure message was sent using the electronic messaging function of CEHRT to the patient (or the patient-authorized representative), or in response to a secure message sent by the patient (or the patient authorized representative), during the performance period.	Up to 10 Points	Numerator/ Denominator

(continued on next page)

By achieving these five Base objectives, you can earn half of the points available for this category: 50 out of 100, which translates to 12.5 of the 25 percent contribution to the Final MIPS score.

To build on that score, clinicians would need to show that they have achieved performance in any of the eight objectives included in the Performance Points outlined below (Table 3-15). It is not mandatory to report on any of these objectives. Instead, clinicians can focus on the ones that are

TABLE 3-15. 2015 Edition Certified EHR Technology Performance Point Requirements (continued)

2015 Edition CEHRT Performance Points				
Objective	Measure	Description	Performance Score	Reporting Requirement
Health Information Exchange	Send Summary of Care	For at least one transition of care or referral, the MIPS-eligible clinician that transitions or refers his patient to another setting of care or health care clinician—(1) creates a summary of care record using CEHRT; and (2) electronically exchanges the summary of care record.	Up to 10 Points	Numerator/ Denominator
Health Information Exchange	Request/ Accept Summary of Care	In at least one transition of care or referral received or patient encounter in which the MIPS-eligible clinician has never before encountered the patient, the MIPS-eligible clinician receives or retrieves and incorporates into the patient's record an electronic summary of care document.	Up to 10 Points	Numerator/ Denominator
Health Information Exchange	Clinical Information Reconciliation	For at least one transition of care or referral received or patient encounter in which the MIPS-eligible clinician has never before encountered the patient, the MIPS-eligible clinician performs clinical information reconciliation. The MIPS-eligible clinician must implement clinical information reconciliation for the following three clinical information sets: (1) Medication. Review of the patient's medication, including the name, dosage, frequency, and route of each medication. (2) Medication Allergy. Review of the patient's known medication allergies. (3) Current Problem List. Review of the patient's current and active diagnoses.	Up to 10 Points	Numerator/ Denominator
Public Health and Clinical Data Registry Reporting	Immunization Registry Reporting	The MIPS-eligible clinician is in active engagement with a public health agency to submit immunization data and receive immunization forecasts and histories from the public health immunization registry/immunization information system (IIS).	0 or 10 Points	Yes/No Statement

meaningful to them or relatively easy to achieve. Offering this level of flexibility to clinicians allows them to reach the full category score through a path of their own choosing.

There are a total of 90 points available in the Performance section, which if all available points were earned, would give a clinician 140 category points. It's important to know that CMS caps the aggregate score at 100.

This next section includes important definitions and "additional information" that is taken directly from the ACI measures specification sheets for each of these Performance objectives.

Provide Patient Access: Keen eyes will notice that this objective was also included in the Base points. In the Base section, CMS is only interested in whether this objective was met *one time*. In the Performance section, CMS takes into account the performance rate for the entire reporting period.

Patient Education:

Patient-Specific Education Resources Identified by CEHRT—Resources or a topic area of resources identified through logic built into certified EHR technology, which evaluates information about the patient and suggests education resources that would be of value to the patient.

Paper-based actions are not included in the numerator and denominator. MIPS-eligible clinicians may still provide paper-based educational materials for their patients, but are not allowed to include them in the measure calculations.

View, Download, Transmit:

API or Application Programming Interface—A set of programming protocols established for multiple purposes. APIs may be enabled by a health care provider or health care provider organization to provide patients with access to their health information through a third-party application with more flexibility than is often found in many current "patient portals."

View—The patient (or authorized representative) accessing their health information online.

Download—The movement of information from online to physical electronic media.

Transmission—This may be any means of electronic transmission according to any transport standard(s) (e.g., SMTP, FTP, REST, SOAP, etc.). However, the relocation of physical electronic media (e.g. USB or CD) does not qualify as transmission.

Unique Patient—If a patient is seen by a MIPS-eligible clinician more than once during the MIPS performance period, then for purposes of measurement, that patient is only counted once in the denominator for the measure. All the measures relying on the term "unique patient" relate to what is contained in the patient's medical record. Not all of this information will need to be updated or even be required by the MIPS-eligible clinician at every patient encounter. This is especially true for patients whose encounter frequency is such that they would see the same MIPS-eligible clinician multiple times in the same MIPS performance period.

There are four actions a patient might take as part of the measure.
1. View their information.
2. Download their information.

3. Transmit their information to a third party.
4. Access their information through an API.

These actions may overlap, but an MIPS-eligible clinician is able to count any and all actions in the single numerator. Therefore, an MIPS-eligible clinician may meet a combined threshold for VDT and API actions, or if her technology functions overlap, then any view, download, transmit, or API actions taken by the patient using CEHRT would count toward the threshold.

In order to meet this measure, the following information must be made available to patients electronically:

• Patient name
• Provider's name and office contact information
• Current and past problem list
• Procedures of Laboratory test results
• Current medication list and medication history
• Current medication allergy list and medication allergy history
• Vital signs (height, weight, blood pressure, BMI, growth charts)
• Smoking status
• Demographic information (preferred language, sex, race, ethnicity, date of birth)
• Care plan field(s), including goals and instructions
• Any known care team members including the primary care provider (PCP) of record

Secure Messaging:

Secure Message—Any electronic communication between an MIPS-eligible clinician and patient that ensures only those parties can access the communication. This electronic message could be email or the electronic messaging function of a PHR, an online patient portal, or any other electronic means.

The Secure Messaging measure under the Advancing Care Information performance category requires that a secure message be sent using the electronic messaging function of CEHRT to the patient (or the patient-authorized representative), or in response to a secure message sent by the patient (or the patient-authorized representative).

The measure includes MIPS-eligible clinician-initiated communications (when an MIPS-eligible clinician sends a message to a patient or the patient's authorized representatives), and clinician-to-clinician communications if the patient is included. A MIPS-eligible clinician can only count messages in the numerator when the MIPS-eligible clinician participates in the communication (e.g., any patient-initiated communication only if the MIPS-eligible clinician responds to the patient.) Note: MIPS-eligible clinicians are not required to respond to every message received if a response is not needed.

Patient Generated Health Data:

Patient-Generated Health Data—Data generated by a patient or a patient's authorized representative.

Data from a Non-Clinical Setting—This includes, but is not limited to, social service data, data generated by a patient or a patient's authorized representative, advance directives, medical device data, home health monitoring data, and fitness monitor data.

Unique Patient—If a patient is seen by a MIPS-eligible clinician more than once during the MIPS performance period, then for purposes of measurement, that patient is only counted once in the denominator for the measure. All the measures relying on the term "unique patient" relate to what is contained in the patient's medical record. Not all of this information will need to be updated or even be needed by the MIPS-eligible clinician at every patient encounter. This is especially true for patients whose encounter frequency is such that they would see the same MIPS-eligible clinician multiple times in the same MIPS performance period.

For the Patient-Generated Health Data measure, the calculation of the numerator incorporates both health data from non-clinical settings, as well as health data generated by the patient.

For the Patient Generated Health Data measure, the types of data that would satisfy the measure are broad. It may include, but is not limited to, social service data, data generated by a patient or a patient's authorized representative, advance directives, medical device data, home health monitoring data, and fitness monitor data. In addition, the sources of data vary and may include mobile applications for tracking health and nutrition, home health devices with tracking capabilities such as scales and blood pressure monitors, wearable devices such as activity trackers or heart monitors, patient-reported outcome data, and other methods of input for patient and non-clinical setting generated health data. (Note: Data related to billing, payment, or other insurance information would not satisfy this measure.)

For the measure, clinicians in non-clinical settings may include, but are not limited to, care providers such as nutritionists, physical therapists, occupational therapists, psychologists, and home health care providers. Other key clinicians in the care team such as behavioral health care providers, may also be included, and CMS encourages clinicians to consider ways in which this measure can incorporate this essential information from the broader care team.

For this measure, we do not specify the manner in which MIPS-eligible clinicians are required to incorporate the data. MIPS-eligible clinicians may work with their EHR developers to establish the methods and processes that work best for their practice and needs. For example, if data provided can be easily incorporated in a structured format or into an existing field within the EHR (such as a C–CDA or care team member reported vital signs or patient reported family health history and demographic information) the MIPS-eligible clinician may elect to do so. Alternately, a MIPS-eligible clinician may maintain isolation between the data and the patient record and instead include the data by other means such as attachments, links, and text references again as best meets their needs.

HIE: Send Summary of Care: See the description from the 2015 Edition Base points section. Information is the same.

HIE: Request/Accept Summary of Care: See the description from the 2015 Edition Base points section. Information is the same.

Clinical Information Reconciliation

Transition of Care—The movement of a patient from one setting of care (e.g., hospital, ambulatory primary care practice, ambulatory, specialty care practice, long-term care, home health, or rehabilitation facility) to another. At a minimum, this includes all transitions of care and referrals that are ordered by the clinician.

Current Problem Lists—At a minimum, a list of current and active diagnoses.

Active/Current Medication List—A list of medications that a given patient is currently taking.

Active/Current Medication Allergy List—A list of medications to which a given patient has known allergies.

Allergy—An exaggerated immune response or reaction to substances that are generally not harmful.

For the measure, the process may include both automated and manual reconciliation to allow the receiving MIPS-eligible clinician to work with both the electronic data provided with any necessary review, and to work directly with the patient to reconcile her health information.

For the measure, if no update is necessary, the process of reconciliation may consist of simply verifying that fact or reviewing a record received on referral and determining that such information is merely duplicative of existing information in the patient record.

Non-medical staff may conduct reconciliation under the direction of the MIPS-eligible clinician so long as the clinician or other credentialed medical staff is responsible and accountable for review of the information and for the assessment of and action on any relevant CDS.

Immunization Registry Reporting

Active Engagement—the MIPS-eligible clinician is in the process of moving towards sending "production data" to a public health agency (PHA) or clinical data registry (CDR), or is sending production data to a PHA or CDR.

Active engagement may be demonstrated in one of the following ways:

Option 1—Completed Registration to Submit Data: The MIPS-eligible clinician registered to submit data with the PHA or, where applicable, the CDR to which the information is being submitted; registration was completed within 60 days after the start of the MIPS performance period; and the MIPS-eligible clinician is awaiting an invitation from the PHA or CDR to begin testing and validation. This option allows MIPS-eligible clinicians to meet the measure when the PHA or the CDR has limited resources to initiate the testing and validation process. MIPS-eligible clinicians who have registered in previous years do not need to submit an additional registration to meet this requirement for each MIPS performance period.

Option 2—Testing and Validation: The MIPS-eligible clinician is in the process of testing and validation of the electronic submission of data. MIPS-eligible clinicians must respond to requests from the PHA or, where applicable, the CDR within 30 days; failure to respond twice within a MIPS performance period would result in that MIPS-eligible clinician not meeting the measure.

Option 3—Production: The MIPS-eligible clinician has completed testing and validation of the electronic submission and is electronically submitting production data to the PHA or CDR.

TABLE 3-16. 2015 Edition certified EHR technology Performance Point Requirements

2015 Edition CEHRT Bonus Points				
Objective	Measure	Description	Performance Score	Reporting Requirement
Public Health and Clinical Data Registry Reporting	Syndromic Surveillance Reporting	The MIPS-eligible clinician is in active engagement with a public health agency to submit syndromic surveillance data.	5 Points	Yes/No Statement
Public Health and Clinical Data Registry Reporting	Clinical Data Registry Reporting	The MIPS-eligible clinician is in active engagement to submit data to a clinical data registry.	5 Points	Yes/No Statement
Public Health and Clinical Data Registry Reporting	Electronic Case Reporting	The MIPS-eligible clinician is in active engagement with a public health agency to electronically submit case reporting of reportable conditions.	5 Points	Yes/No Statement
Public Health and Clinical Data Registry Reporting	Public Health Registry Reporting	The MIPS-eligible clinician is in active engagement with a public health agency to submit data to public health registries.	5 Points	Yes/No Statement
Report Improvement Activities using CEHRT		The MIPS-eligible clinician attests to have submitted an eligible Improvement Activity using certified EHR technology	10 Points	Yes/No Statement
Report Using Only 2015 Edition CEHRT		The MIPS-eligible clinician attests to using only 2015 Edition certified EHR technology	10 Points	Based on Measures Submitted

Production Data—Refers to data generated through clinical processes involving patient care, and it is used to distinguish between data and "test data," which may be submitted for the purposes of enrolling in and testing electronic data transfers.

MIPS-eligible clinicians may choose to report the Immunization Registry Reporting measure to increase their Advancing Care Information performance score. The Advancing Care Information bonus score will only be awarded for reporting to additional public health or clinical data registries (Table 3-16).

For the measure, an MIPS-eligible clinician's health IT system may layer additional information on the immunization history and forecast, and *still* successfully meet this measure.

Bi-directionality provides that certified health IT must be able to receive and display a consolidated immunization history and forecast in addition to sending the immunization record.

MIPS-eligible clinicians who have previously registered, tested, or begun ongoing submission of data to registry do not need to "restart" the process. The MIPS-eligible clinician may simply attest to the active engagement option that most closely reflects their current status.

CMS has developed a centralized repository for PHA and CDR reporting. The collected data is posted on the EHR Incentive Programs website at https://www.cms.gov/Regulations-and-Guidance/Legislation/EHRIncentivePrograms/CentralizedRepository-.html.

Syndromic Surveillance Reporting

Active Engagement—the MIPS-eligible clinician is in the process of moving towards sending "production data" to a public health agency (PHA) or clinical data registry (CDR), or is sending production data to a PHA or CDR.

Active engagement may be demonstrated in one of the following ways:

Option 1—Completed Registration to Submit Data: The MIPS-eligible clinician registered to submit data with the PHA or, where applicable, the CDR to which the information is being submitted; registration was completed within 60 days after the start of the MIPS performance period; and the MIPS-eligible clinician is awaiting an invitation from the PHA or CDR to begin testing and validation. This option allows MIPS-eligible clinicians to meet the measure when the PHA or the CDR has limited resources to initiate the testing and validation process. MIPS-eligible clinicians who have registered in previous years are not required to submit an additional registration to meet this requirement for each MIPS performance period.

Option 2—Testing and Validation: The MIPS-eligible clinician is in the process of testing and validation of the electronic submission of data. MIPS-eligible clinicians must respond to requests from the PHA or, where applicable, the CDR within 30 days; failure to respond twice within a MIPS performance period would result in that MIPS-eligible clinician not achieving the measure.

Option 3—Production: The MIPS-eligible clinician has completed testing and validation of the electronic submission and is electronically submitting production data to the PHA or CDR.

Production Data—Refers to data generated through clinical processes involving patient care, and it is used to distinguish between data and "test data," which may be submitted for the purposes of enrolling in and testing electronic data transfers.

Active engagement with a public health and clinical data registry will earn the MIPS-eligible clinician a bonus of five percentage points. MIPS-eligible clinicians may also report to the one or more of the following measures to earn the bonus score of five percentage points: clinical data registry reporting, electronic case reporting, or public health registry reporting.

MIPS-eligible clinicians who have previously registered, tested, or begun ongoing submission of data to a registry do not need to "restart" the process. The MIPS-eligible clinician may simply attest to the active engagement option that most closely reflects her current status.

Electronic Case Reporting—Same information as Syndromic Surveillance above.

Public Health Registry Reporting—Same as Syndromic Surveillance above, except with this additional information:

Public Health Registry is administered by, or on behalf of, a local, state, territorial, or national public health agency that collects data for public health purposes.

Clinical Data Registry Reporting—Same as above, except with this additional information:

CDRs are administered by, or on behalf of, other non-public health agency entities. They provide information that can inform patients and their health care providers on the best course of treatment and care improvements, and can support specialty reporting by developing reporting for areas not usually covered by public health agencies but that are important to a specialist's provision of care. CDRs can also be used to monitor health care quality and resource use.

The definition of jurisdiction is general, and the scope may be local, state, regional, or at the national level. The definition will be dependent on the type of registry to which the provider is reporting. A registry that is "borderless" would be considered a registry at the national level and would be included for purposes of this measure.

Report Improvement Activities Using Certified EHR Technology

There is a subset of Improvement Activities that award you bonus points in the ACI category, specifically, when an Improvement Activity uses Certified EHR to achieve it. When choosing your Improvement Activities, consider which of these measures will afford you a 10-point bonus in the ACI category.

Clinicians will need to perform an annual Security Risk Assessment (SRA) to keep protected health information that is created or maintained by the EHR private and secure. Failure to complete this task alone would result in a Base Score of zero regardless of the clinician's adherence to any of the other ACI objectives. I emphasize this because, to date, the SRA is the number one reason clinicians fail audits.

Using 2015 Edition CEHRT for the Entire Reporting Period

CMS will offer a one-time bonus of 10 percentage points under the ACI performance category for MIPS-eligible clinicians who, using only 2015 Edition certified HER technology, report the ACI objectives and measures for the performance period in 2018.

Option 3—2014/2015 Combo Edition

It may turn out that some clinicians will be on 2014 Edition technology for part of the year and 2015 Edition technology for the remainder. These clinicians may choose to report the objectives and measures for either Edition, as long as they have the technologies to support each measure selected.

Understanding ACI Scoring

Now that we've discussed the objectives in detail, let's take a moment to understand, in depth, how CMS scores the ACI category.

Base Score

First, to receive *any* score within the ACI performance category, an MIPS-eligible clinician must meet each of the Base Score requirements, unless she qualifies for an exclusion.

This process begins with achieving the Protect Patient Health Information objective and measure. Clinicians will need to perform an annual Security Risk Assessment (SRA) to keep protected health information that is created or maintained by the EHR private and secure. Failure to complete this task alone would result in a Base Score of zero regardless of the clinician's adherence to any of the other ACI objectives. I emphasize this because, to date, the SRA is the number one reason clinicians fail audits.

Next, there must be a minimum of at least "1" in the numerator for the other required EHR-based objectives:

- e-Prescribing*
- Provide Patient Access
- HIE: Send Summary of Care*
- HIE: Request/Accept Summary of Care* (*2015 Edition only*)
  * Exclusions are available to clinicians who meet the criteria.

A clinician or group that accomplishes these tasks will receive half of the points available for this category. Remember, there are a total of 25 MIPS points available for this performance category and 100 ACI category points, so completing the above criteria is worth 12.5 MIPS points or 50 ACI category points.

Performance Score

The Performance Score builds upon the Base Score and is derived from the clinician's or group's performance rate (i.e. numerator/denominator) for each measure reported from the performance score options. A performance rate between 1 to 10 percent would earn one percentage point and a rate between 11 to 20 percent would earn two percentage points and so on.

For example, if the clinician reports a numerator/denominator of 85/100 for the Patient Education measure, the performance rate would be 85 percent and the clinician would earn nine percentage points toward her performance score for the ACI category.

For both 2014 and 2015 Edition technologies, MIPS-eligible clinicians have the ability to earn up to 90 percentage points if they report all measures in the performance score (Table 3-17).

TABLE 3-17. ACI Deciles for Performance Score

ACI Deciles for Performance Score	
Performance Rate	Points Earned
1-10 %	1
11-20 %	2
21-30 %	3
31-40 %	4
41-50 %	5
51-60 %	6
61-70 %	7
71-80 %	8
81-90 %	9
91-100 %	10

Since the Public Health and Clinical Data Registry Reporting objective does not have a numerator/denominator to calculate the performance rate, CMS will award zero or 10 percentage points (0 percent for a "no" response, 10 percent for a "yes" response) for the Immunization Registry Reporting measure.

Take note that two of the measures in the base score are *not* included in the performance score. This means that a clinician will not earn additional points under the performance score for reporting them. The measures are:
• Protect Patient Health Information
• e-Prescribing

TABLE 3-18. Improvement Activities Eligible for ACI Bonus

	Improvement Activity	Activity ID#	Weight	Related ACI Measure(s)
1	Provide 24/7 access to eligible clinicians or groups who have real-time access to patient's medical record.	IA_EPA_1	High	Provide Patient Access Secure Messaging Send a Summary of Care Request/Accept Summary of Care
2	Anticoagulant management improvements	IA_PM_2	High	Provide Patient Access Patient-Specific Education View, Download, Transmit Secure Messaging Patient Generated Health Data or Data from Non- Clinical Setting Send a Summary of Care Request/ Accept Summary of Care Care Clinical Information Reconciliation Exchange Clinical Decision Support (CEHRT Function Only)
3	Glycemic management services	IA_PM_4	High	Patient Generated Health Data Clinical Information Reconciliation Clinical Decision Support, CCDS, Family Health History (CEHRT functions only)

(continued on next page)

Bonus Points

As mentioned previously, there are several ways to earn bonus points in the ACI category.

Certain improvement activities from the Improvement Activities performance category can be tied to objectives, measures, and EHR functions of the ACI category and therefore qualify for a bonus in the ACI category.

Table 3-18, Improvement Activities Eligible for ACI Bonus, provides a complete list of the improvement activities that are eligible for the ACI performance category bonus. These activities can be tied to the objectives, measures, and CEHRT functionality of the ACI performance category and would thus qualify for the bonus in the Advancing Care Information performance category if they are reported using CEHRT.

CMS will award a 10 percent bonus in the ACI performance category if an MIPS-eligible clinician attests to completing at least one of the improvement activities in Table 3-18. Also, the weight of the improvement activity (high or medium) will have no bearing on the bonus awarded in the ACI performance category.

Additionally, active engagement with a public health or clinical data registry to meet any other measure associated with the Public Health and

TABLE 3-18. Improvement Activities Eligible for ACI Bonus (continued)

	Improvement Activity	Activity ID#	Weight	Related ACI Measure(s)
4	Chronic care and preventative care management for empaneled patients	IA_PM_13	Medium	Provide Patient Access Patient-Specific Education View, Download, Transmit Secure Messaging Patient Generated Health Data or Data from Non-Clinical Setting Send A Summary of Care Request/Accept Summary of care Clinical Information Reconciliation Clinical Decision Support, Family Health History (CEHRT functions only)
5	Implementation of methodologies for improvements in longitudinal care management for high risk patients	IA_PM_14	Medium	Provide Patient Access Patient-Specific Education Patient Generated Health Data or Data from Non-clinical Settings Send A Summary of Care Request/Accept Summary of Care Clinical information reconciliation Clinical Decision Support, CCDS, Family Health History, Patient List (CEHRT functions only)
6	Implementation of episodic care management practice improvements	IA_PM_15	Medium	Send A Summary of Care Request/ Accept Summary of Care Clinical Information Reconciliation
7	Implementation of medication management practice improvements	IA_PM_16	Medium	Clinical Information Reconciliation Clinical Decision Support, Computerized Physician Order Entry Electronic Prescribing (CEHRT functions only)
8	Implementation or use of specialist reports back to referring clinician or group to close referral loop	IA_CC_1	Medium	Send A Summary of Care Request/Accept Summary of Care Clinical Information Reconciliation
9	Implementation of documentation improvements for practice/process improvements	IA_CC_8	Medium	Secure Messaging Send a Summary of Care Request/Accept Summary of Care Clinical Information Reconciliation

(continued on next page)

Clinical Data Registry Reporting objective will earn the MIPS-eligible clinician a bonus of 10 points. Note that clinicians are not required to report the Immunization Registry Reporting measure in order to earn the 10 bonus points for reporting to one or more additional registries.

Lastly, clinicians who only use 2015 Edition EHR technology in 2018 qualify for a one-time bonus of 10 percentage points.

TABLE 3-18. Improvement Activities Eligible for ACI Bonus (continued)

	Improvement Activity	Activity ID#	Weight	Related ACI Measure(s)
10	Implementation of practices/processes for developing regular individual care plans	IA_CC_9	Medium	Provide Patient Access (formerly Patient Access) View, Download, Transmit Secure Messaging Patient Generated Health Data or Data from Non- Clinical Setting
11	Practice improvements for bilateral exchange of patient information	IA_CC_13	Medium	Send A Summary of Care Request/ Accept Summary of Care Clinical Information Reconciliation
12	Use of certified EHR to capture patient reported outcomes	IA_BE-1	Medium	Provide Patient Access Patient-specific Education Care Coordination through Patient Engagement
13	Engagement of patients through implementation of improvements in patient portal	IA_BE_14	Medium	Provide Patient Access Patient-specific Education
14	Engagement of patients, family and caregivers in developing a plan of care	IA_BE_15	Medium	Provide Patient Access Patient-specific Education View, Download, Transmit (Patient Action) Secure Messaging
15	Use of decision support and standardized treatment protocols	IA_PSPA_16	Medium	Clinical Decision Support (CEHRT function only)
16	Leveraging a QCDR to standardize processes for screening			Patient Generated Health Date or Data from a Non-Clinical Setting Public Health and Clinical Data Registry Reporting
17	Implementation of integrated PCBH model	IA_BMH_7	High	Provide Patient Access Patient-Specific Education View, Download, Transmit Secure Messaging Patient Generated Health Data or Data from Non-clinical Setting
18	Electronic Health Record Enhancements for BH data capture	IA_BMH_8	Medium	Patient Generated Health Data or Data from Non-clinical Setting Send A Summary of Care Request/ Accept Summary of Care Clinical Information Reconciliation
19	Promote use of patient-reported outcome tools	IA_AHE_3	High	Public Health Registry Reporting Clinical Data Registry Reporting Patient-Generated Health Data
20	Perioperative Surgical Home (PSH) care coordination	IA_CC_15	Medium	Send a Summary of Care Request/Accept Summary of Care Clinical Information Reconciliation Health Information Exchange

(continued on next page)

TABLE 3-18. Improvement Activities Eligible for ACI Bonus (continued)

	Improvement Activity	Activity ID#	Weight	Related ACI Measure(s)
21	Primary care physician and behavioral health bilateral electronic exchange of information for shared patients	IA_CC_16	Medium	Send a Summary of Care Request/Accept Summary of Care
22	Provide clinical-community linkages	IA_PM_18	Medium	Provide Patient Access Patient-Specific Education Patient-Generated Health Data
23	Glycemic screening services	IA_PM_19	Medium	Patient-Specific Education Patient-Generated Health Data
24	Glycemic referring services	IA_PM_20	Medium	Patient-Specific Education Patient-Generated Health Data
25	Advance care planning	IA_PM_21	Medium	Patient-Specific Education Patient-Generated Health Data
26	Communication of unscheduled visit for adverse drug event and nature of event	IA_PSPA_26	Medium	Secure Messaging Send a Summary of Care Request/Accept Summary of Care
27	Consulting AUC using clinical decision support when ordering advanced diagnostic imaging	IA_PSPA_28	Medium	Clinical Decision Support (CEHRT function only)

TABLE 3-19. Scoring the ACI Category

Base Score	Performance Score	Bonus Points (Public Health or Clinical Registry)	Bonus Points (Improvement Activities through CEHRT)	Bonus Points (2015 Edition CEHRT)	ACI Performance Score
50 points	**Up to 90 points**	**Up to 10 points**	**Up to 10 points**	**Up to 10 percentage points**	**100+ points** (capped at 100)
Awarded for providing numerator/denominator or "yes" statement for each required objective and measure	Earned through performance rates on seven (2014 Edition) or nine (2015 Edition) objectives and measures	By reporting to public health and clinical data registries beyond the Immunization Registry Reporting measure	By reporting an Improvement Activity using certified EHR technology	By only using 2015 Edition certified EHR technology for the full reporting period	Scoring 100 points or more in the ACI category will earn full credit (25%) of the MIPS Score

Composite Score

In total, when the Base score, Performance score, and Bonus score are compiled, clinicians have the potential to earn up to 160 percentage points with the 2014 Edition EHR or up to 170 percentage points with the 2015 Edition EHR in the ACI performance category (Table 3-19). Friendly reminder: the category score will be capped at 100 percentage points.

Final ACI category scores will then be converted to reflect up to 25 MIPS points.

2014 Edition Scoring Example (Tables 3-20 and 3-21)

TABLE 3-20. 2014 Edition certified EHR technology Scoring Example

2014 CEHRT Reporting Option for 2018 Performance Year					
Base Score*	**Objective**	**Measure**	**Y/N or Num/Den**	**Performance Score**	**Points Available**
* Failure to meet the base score requirements will result in a zero in the ACI category (ECs will score 0 or 50) ** Exclusions apply	**Protect Patient Information**	SRA	Y/N	0	50
	E-prescribing**	E-prescribing	Num/Den, min. 1/1	0	
	Patient Electronic Access	Provide Patient Access	Num/Den, min. 1/1	See below.	
	Health Info Exchange**	Send Summary of Care	Num/Den, min. 1/1	See below.	
Performance Score	**Objective**	**Measure**	**Y/N or Num/Den**	**Performance Score**	**Points Available**
	Patient Electronic Access	Provide Patient Access	Num/Den, min. 1/1	Up to 20%	90
		VDT	Num/Den, min. 1/1	Up to 10%	
	Patient Education	Patient Education	Num/Den, min. 1/1	Up to 10%	
	Secure Messaging	Secure Messaging	Num/Den, min. 1/1	Up to 10%	
	Health Info Exchange	Send Summary of Care	Num/Den, min. 1/1	Up to 20%	
	Medication Reconciliation	Medication reconciliation	Num/Den, min. 1/1	Up to 10%	
	Public Health	Immunization Registry	Y/N	0 or 10%	
Bonus Points					
	Public Health Registry Reporting	Syndromic Surveillance Reporting	Y/N	10%	20
		Public Health Registry Reporting	Y/N		
	Completed Improvement Activity Using CEHRT		Y/N	10%	
Total Points (Capped at 100)					160

TABLE 3-21. 2014 Edition certified EHR technology Scorecard Example for an Individual Clinician

Account #	Summary	Avail. Pts	Jan
#	Base Points Earned	0 or 50	50
Practice Name	Performance Points Earned	90	31
ABC Practice	Bonus Points Earned	20	10
EC Name	Total ACI Points Earned	160	91
Dr. C			
NPI	ACI SCORE	25	23
123456789			

Base Score

Objective	Measure		Jan
Protect Patient Information	SRA		y
E-prescribing	E-prescribing		y
Patient Electronic Access	Provide Patient Access		y
Health Info Exchange	Send Summary of Care		y

Performance Score

Objective	Measure		Jan
Patient Electronic Access	Provide Patient Access	Den	30
		%	66%
	VDT	Den	5
		%	1%
Patient Education	Patient Education	Den	90
		%	58%
Secure Messaging	Secure Messaging	Den	5
		%	5%
Health Info Exchange	Send Summary of Care	Den	10
		%	0%
Medication Reconciliation	Medication reconciliation	Den	50
		%	89%
Public Health	Immunization Registry		n

Bonus Score

Objective	Measure		Jan
Public Health Registry Reporting	Syndromic Surveillance Reporting		n
	Public Health Registry Reporting		n
Completed Improvement Activity Using CEHRT			y

2015 Edition Scoring Example (Tables 3-22 and 3-23)

TABLE 3-22. 2015 Edition certified EHR technology Scoring Example

2015 CEHRT Reporting Option for 2017 Transition Year					
Base Score*	**Objective**	**Measure**	**Y/N or Num/Den**	**Performance Score**	**Points Available**
* Failure to meet the base score requirements will result in a zero in the ACI category (ECs will score 0 or 50) ** Exclusions apply	**Protect Patient Information**	SRA	Y/N	0	50
	E-prescribing**	E-prescribing	Num/Den, min. 1/1	0	
	Provide Electronic Access	Provide Patient Access	Num/Den, min. 1/1	See below.	
	Health Information Exchange**	Send Summary of Care	Num/Den, min. 1/1	See below.	
		Request/Accept Summary of Care	Num/Den, min. 1/1	See below.	
Performance Score	**Objective**	**Measure**	**Y/N or Num/Den**	**Performance Score**	**Points Available**
	Patient Electronic Access	Provide Patient Access	Num/Den, min. 1/1	Up to 10%	90
		Patient Education	Num/Den, min. 1/1	Up to 10%	
	Coordination of Care through Patient Engagement	VDT	Num/Den, min. 1/1	Up to 10%	
		Secure Messaging	Num/Den, min. 1/1	Up to 10%	
		Patient Generated Health Data	Num/Den, min. 1/1	Up to 10%	
	Health Information Exchange	Send Summary of Care	Num/Den, min. 1/1	Up to 10%	
		Request/Accept Summary of Care	Num/Den, min. 1/1	Up to 10%	
		Clinical Information Reconciliation	Num/Den, min. 1/1	Up to 10%	
	Public Health	Immunization Registry	Y/N	0 or 10%	
Bonus Score	**Objective**	**Measure**	**Y/N or Num/Den**	**Performance Score**	**Points Available**
	Public Health and Clinical Data Registry Reporting	Syndromic Surveillance Reporting	Y/N	10%	30
		Electronic Case Reporting	Y/N		
		Public Health Registry Reporting	Y/N		
		Clinical Data Registry Reporting	Y/N		
	Report Improvement Activities Using CEHRT		Y/N	10%	
	Report Using only 2015 Edition CEHRT		Y/N	10%	
Total Points (Capped at 100)					170

TABLE 3-23. 2015 Edition certified EHR technology Scorecard Example for an Individual Clinician

Account #	Summary	Avail. Pts		Jan
#	Base Points Earned	0 or 50		50
Practice Name	Performance Points Earned	90		32
ABC Practice	Bonus Points Earned	30		20
EC Name	Total ACI Points Earned	170		102
Dr. C				
NPI	**ACI SCORE**	**25**		**25**
123456789				

Base Score	Objective	Measure		Jan
	Protect Patient Information	SRA		Y
	E-prescribing	E-prescribing		Y
	Patient Electronic Access	Provide Patient Access		Y
	Health Info Exchange	Send Summary of Care		Y
		Request/Accept Summary of Care		Y

Performance Score	Objective	Measure		Jan
	Patient Electronic Access	Provide Patient Access	Den	134
			%	66%
		Patient Education	Den	137
			%	51%
	Coordination of Care through Patient Engagement	VDT	Den	134
			%	2%
		Secure Messaging	Den	134
			%	0%
		Patient Generated Health Data	Den	2
			%	0%
	Health Info Exchange	Send Summary of Care	Den	13
			%	5%
		Request/Accept Summary of Care	Den	5%
			%	0%
		Clinical Information Reconciliation	Den	47%
			%	92%
	Public Health	Immunization Registry		N

Bonus Score	Objective	Measure		Jan
	Public Health Registry Reporting	Syndromic Surveillance Reporting		N
		Electronic Case Reporting		N
		Clinical Data Registry Reporting		N
		Public Health Registry Reporting		Y
	Report Improvement Activities Using CEHRT			N
	Report ACI Using only 2015 CEHRT			Y

Keys to Success

- Don't forget about the required Security Risk Analysis—it's the only Base objective that is not tracked within your EHR. Many practices accomplish this task with their IT vendor or through a third party vendor or consultant.
- The Health Information Exchange component can be tricky—some EHRs have Direct Mail built-in to their systems. Other EHRs use a third party vendor (such as Updox) and integrate the functionality. And 2014 Edition EHRs can only send and receive information (i.e. they cannot request it), whereas 2015 Edition EHRs can send, receive, and also request a patient record be sent to them. Make sure you understand the capabilities of your EHR. Call your vendor to get help!
- Since Providing Patient Access can earn up to 20 points in the 2014 Edition option, one way to maintain consistently high performance rates in this objective is to configure the EHR to automatically enroll and register all new patients with an account to access the patient portal.
- The Patient-Generated Health Data is brand new for everyone, since the functionality can only be utilized in 2015 Edition EHRs. Patient-generated data likely brings to mind Fitbits, wearables, and other smart devices, but it can take the form of something as simple as a patient being able to correct erroneous information contained in their electronic health record. It may also encompass remote monitoring of cancer and diabetes patients or those recovering from surgery.
- Prepare for an audit as you accomplish tasks in this category by building up a book of evidence. This would include screenshots, letters from your vendor, confirmation emails from any registries, and more.

Resources

- https://qpp.cms.gov/measures/aci
- Download the full ACI measure specifications: https://www.cms.gov/Medicare/Quality-Payment-Program/Resource-Library/2018-Resources.html
- Security Risk Analysis Tip Sheet: https://www.cms.gov/Regulations-and-Guidance/Legislation/EHRIncentivePrograms/Downloads/2016_SecurityRiskAnalysis.pdf
- Your EHR's resource library should detail the workflows required to accomplish each objective within the system.

Lessons Learned from the Field

Lesson 1: Health Information Exchange

Across the board in 2017, clinicians struggled with this objective. For many, the introduction of new terminology was confusing.

- Health Information Exchange
- HIPS Address
- Direct Mail Address

When we asked if they had any of these, my team and I would get blank stares and start to hear crickets.

The first hurdle of HIE is getting your HIPAA-secure email set up correctly within your EHR. In many cases, this requires contacting your EHR vendor for instructions and sometimes paying their fee associated with accessing this feature.

Since the objective requires the "exchange" of information, the second hurdle is finding others in your referral network who are also set up correctly and using this feature of their EHR.

Once the configurations are in place, an exchange can take place.

Lesson 2: EHR Licensing Issues

Prior to MIPS, mid-level clinicians such as Nurse Practitioners (NPs) and Physician Assistants (Pas) did not need reports verifying their use of the EHR. However, since they are now considered eligible clinicians, EHRs must report more data for them.

In some cases, EHR vendors are charging hefty annual fees—I've seen as much as $7,000 per clinician—just to gain access to their data. A practice with one

doctor, two PAs, and two NPs would see their annual maintenance fee increase by $28,000. Considering how much is billed under these clinicians, in some cases this fee may be greater than any penalty they would incur.

Lesson 3: Utilize the Patient Portal

In many ways, the patient portal is laying the groundwork for interoperability and sharing health data. It is the place where patients can see their health records, update their social and family history, view and update their medications, and even send messages directly to their doctor. Some patient portals serve as a place to learn more about their specific conditions.

In a growing number of ways, it is the launching pad for engaging patients in their health and providing them with more transparency. Patient portals also offer the convenience of being able to share this important information with other health providers in their network, with their caregivers, or to just review for themselves while having easy access for any future needs.

Some practices still struggle with getting their patients to visit the portal, claiming that their patients are too old for technology or that they just aren't interested. While there may be some truth to this, we also know that the aging population is becoming more and more comfortable with technology. The culture is shifting and there are plenty of grandmas with iPhones, iPads, and Kindles, for example.

Practices that consistently provide their patients with online access to their health information are positioned to do well in the ACI category.

Measuring cost is quite possibly the most integral part of measuring value and also probably the most difficult area to wrap your head around. It is so important, in fact, that CMS wrote into the MACRA law that Cost would eventually account for 30 percent of the total MIPS score, beginning with the 2019 performance year. To build up to that ratio and offer clinicians an opportunity to better understand how this category is measured, CMS provided clinicians a "free pass" in the 2017 Transition Year, where cost data was collected through administrative claims for Medicare patients that were attributed to an individual clinician or group, but the information was not used to determine any part of the MIPS score.

However, the Cost category was finalized to contribute 10 percent of the Final Score for the 2018 performance year and will grow again in the 2019 performance year to reflect the full 30 percent weight (Figure 3-11).

COST

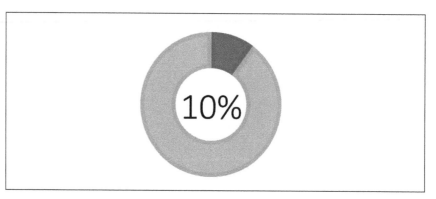

FIGURE 3-11. 2018 Cost Weight

The Cost category is built from the foundations laid by the Value-based Modifier (VM) program, which was originally introduced as part of the Patient Protection and Affordable Care Act (also known as ACA or "Obamacare"), passed in 2010. The VM was not on the radar of most small and solo practitioners for some time because, for its first two years, it only applied to groups with more than 10 providers. In 2015, VM scoring was applied to all Medicare providers regardless of practice size.

Measuring cost is quite possibly the most integral part of measuring value and also probably the most difficult area to wrap your head around. It is so important, in fact, that CMS wrote into the MACRA law that Cost would eventually account for 30 percent of the total MIPS score, beginning with the 2019 performance year. To build up to that ratio and offer clinicians an opportunity to better understand how this category is measured, CMS provided clinicians a "free pass" in the 2017 Transition Year, where cost data was collected through administrative claims for Medicare patients that were attributed to an individual clinician or group, but the information was not used to determine any part of the MIPS score.

However, the Cost category was finalized to contribute 10 percent of the Final Score for the 2018 performance year and will grow again in the 2019 performance year to reflect the full 30 percent weight (Figure 3-11).

Like the Quality category, the Cost category's reporting period will reflect the full calendar year for 2018 and will continue to do so going forward. And unlike the Quality category, benchmarks are *not* based on a previous year. Instead, clinician performance will be compared against the performance of other MIPS-eligible clinicians and groups during the current performance period.

The Cost category score for 2018 will be calculated by taking the average of two measures:
- Medicare Spending Per Beneficiary (MSPB)
- Total Per Capita Cost for all attributed beneficiaries

Both of these measures were used in the VM program as well as in the MIPS Transition year.

If for some reason, only one of these measures can be scored, the score for that measure will serve as the performance category score.

No additional information is required to be submitted to CMS for the Cost performance category, since each individual MIPS-eligible clinician's and group's cost performance will be calculated using administrative claims data if they meet the case minimum of attributed patients.

As Figure 3-12 shows, each cost measure has a different case minimum requirement.
- MSPB case minimum = 35
- Total Per Capita Cost for all attributed beneficiaries = 20

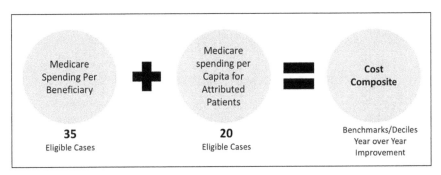

FIGURE 3-12. Case Minimum for Cost Category

These measures are defined as follows:

Medicare Spending Per Beneficiary (MSPB)

This measure assesses Medicare Part A and B costs incurred during an episode, where an episode includes the dates falling between three days prior to an Inpatient Prospective Payment System (IPPS) hospital admission (also referred to as an "index admission") and 30 days after hospital discharge.

The MSPB measure evaluates the observed cost of episodes compared to their expected costs.

For the MSPB measure:
- Clinicians who do not see patients in the hospital will not be attributed to any episodes and not scored on the measure.

> If for some reason, only one of these measures can be scored, the score for that measure will serve as the performance category score.

- Clinicians must be attributed to at least 35 cases to be scored on this measure.
- Episodes will be attributed to the clinician who provided the plurality of Medicare Part B services to a beneficiary during an index admission.

The numerator for a TIN's specialty-adjusted MSPB Measure is the TIN's average MSPB amount, defined as the sum of standardized, risk-adjusted spending across all of a TIN's eligible episodes divided by the number of episodes for that TIN. This ratio is then multiplied by the national average standardized episode cost.

The denominator for a TIN's MSPB Measures is the specialty-adjusted MSPB expected cost on the national specialty-specific expected cost of the specialties represented by the TIN's eligible clinicians (Figure 3-13).

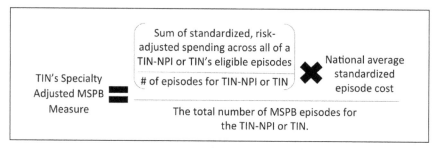

FIGURE 3-13. MSPB Measure Calculation

The beneficiary populations eligible to be included in the MSPB Measure are made up of beneficiaries who were enrolled in both Medicare Parts A and B for the period from 93 days prior to IPPS hospital admission until 30 days after discharge from a short-term acute care hospital stay, where the stay occurs during the period of performance. Defining the population in this manner ensures that each beneficiary's claims record contains sufficient fee-for-service (FFS) data both for measuring spending levels and for risk adjustment purposes.

Only claims for beneficiaries admitted to subsection (d) hospitals* during the period of performance are included in the calculation of the MSPB Measure.

*Subsection (d) hospitals are hospitals in the 50 States and D.C. other than: psychiatric hospitals, rehabilitation hospitals, hospitals whose inpatients are predominantly under 18 years of age, hospitals whose average inpatient length of stay exceeds 25 days, and hospitals involved extensively in treatment for or research on cancer. The claims for inpatient admissions to subsection (d) hospitals are grouped into "stays" by beneficiary, admission date, and provider.

Attribution for MSPB Measure

The Medicare spending per beneficiary (MSPB) follows the existing method of the old value modifier program. It examines the number of services, *computing total allowed charges for Part B care*, during an inpatient stay that is considered an index admission. Note: An index admission is the admission with a principal diagnosis of a specified condition that meets the inclusion/exclusion criteria of a measure. For example, admission for a deep laceration and overnight monitoring would not be included, Admission for Acute Myocardial Infarction (AMI) related to CAD may likely be included.

Each episode is attributed to the one TIN responsible for the plurality of Part B carrier services.

Total Per Capita Cost for All Attributed Beneficiaries

This measure assesses and sums all Medicare Part A and B costs for each attributed beneficiary.

For the Total Per Capita Cost measure:

- Clinicians must have at least 20 unique beneficiaries attributed to them to be scored on this measure.
- Attribution uses a two-step process:

  Step 1: When a patient seeks the bulk of services (based on the number of visits and the cost of those visits) from a provider with a primary care taxonomy designation, the patient is assigned to the TIN as a "Step 1" attribution.

  Primary care taxonomy designations include, but are not limited to, internal medicine, gynecology, family practice, Physician Assistants, and Nurse Practitioners.

  Step 2: When a patient seeks the bulk of services (based on the number of visits and the cost of those visits) from a provider with a specialty taxonomy designation, the patient is assigned to the TIN as a "Step 2" attribution.

  Specialty taxonomy designation is reserved for nearly all specialty care providers.

A Little More About Primary Care Services

Primary care services are defined by the set of services identified by the following Healthcare Common Procedure Coding System (HCPCS)/CPT Codes (Table 3-24).

TABLE 3-24. Procedure Codes that Count as Primary Care Services

HCPCS Codes	Brief Description
99201-99205	New patient, office, or other outpatient visit
99211-99215	Established patient, office, or other outpatient visit
99304-99306	New or established patient, initial nursing facility care
99307-99310	New or established patient, subsequent nursing facility care
99315-99316	New or established patient, discharge day management service
99318	New or established patient, other nursing facility service
99324-99328	New patient, domiciliary, rest home, or custodial care visit
99334-99337	Established patient, domiciliary, rest home, or custodial care visit
99339-99340	Established patient, physician supervision of patient (patient not present) in home, domiciliary, or rest home
99341-99345	New patient, home visit
99347-99350	Established patient, home visit
G0402	Initial Medicare visit
G0438-G0439	Annual wellness visit
G0463	Hospital outpatient clinic visit (Electing Teaching Amendment hospitals only)
99495-99496	Transitional Care Management (TCM) codes
99490	Chronic Care Management (CCM) code

Services billed under CPT codes 99304 through 99318—nursing visits that occur in a skilled nursing facility (SNF), when the claim includes the place of service (POS) 31 modifier—will be excluded from the definition of primary care services.

A Little More About Attribution

In the past, CMS used the VM to attribute Medicare patients to a TIN. Going forward, the plan is to attribute patients and cost measures at the TIN/NPI level for eligible clinicians who report as individuals and at the TIN level for those who elect to participate in MIPS as a group.

MIPS-eligible clinicians that choose to have their performance assessed as a group will first be attributed at the individual TIN/NPI level and then have all cases assigned to the individual TIN/NPIs attributed to the group under which they bill. This alternative would apply one consistent methodology to both groups and individuals, compared to having a methodology that assigns cases using TIN/NPI for assessment at the individual level and another that assigns cases using only TIN for assessment at the group level.

For solo practitioners, this does not present a significant change, but for those who practice in a group, and plan to participate in MIPS as an individual, it does. Since all four performance categories must be assessed the same—as an individual or as a group—this change to the attribution logic is likely to change the attributed cases, which in turn could affect a clinician's performance on cost measures.

For example, a TIN may have one clinician with 10 attributed beneficiaries and another with 12 attributed beneficiaries. If they report as individuals, neither would be scored on the measure. However, if they report as a group, they would receive a score since they reach the 20-case minimum threshold (10 cases + 12 cases = 22 cases).

The "plurality of claims" will be determined by the TIN/NPI for both groups and individuals. However, for individuals, only the MSPB measure attributed to the TIN/NPI would be evaluated. But for groups, the MSPB measure attributed to any TIN/NPI billing under the TIN would be evaluated. For those groups that participate in group reporting through other MIPS performance categories, their cost performance category scores will be determined by aggregating the scores of the individual clinicians within the TIN.

For solo practitioners, this does not present a significant change, but for those who practice in a group, and plan to participate in MIPS as an individual, it does. Since all four performance categories must be assessed the same—as an individual or as a group—this change to the attribution logic is likely to change the attributed cases, which in turn could affect a clinician's performance on cost measures.

Scoring

The Cost category score will be calculated from the Medicare administrative claims. **No additional data submission is required for the 2018 performance year (Figure 3-14).**

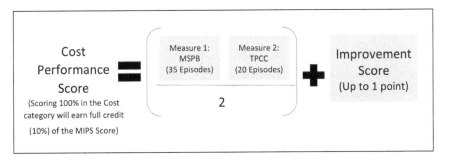

FIGURE 3-14. Scoring the Cost Category

The Cost score will be calculated by comparing performance against benchmarks and then assigning somewhere between zero to 10 points (Figure 3-15).

- The Cost benchmarks will be based on the performance for the same year, unlike the Quality benchmarks that are based on prior years' performance.

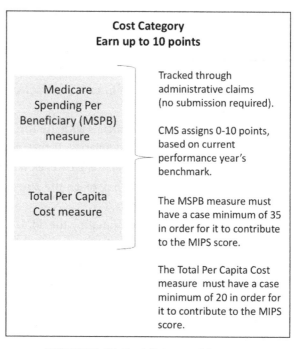

Cost Category
Earn up to 10 points

Medicare Spending Per Beneficiary (MSPB) measure

Tracked through administrative claims (no submission required).

CMS assigns 0-10 points, based on current performance year's benchmark.

Total Per Capita Cost measure

The MSPB measure must have a case minimum of 35 in order for it to contribute to the MIPS score.

The Total Per Capita Cost measure must have a case minimum of 20 in order for it to contribute to the MIPS score.

FIGURE 3-15. Cost Category Measures

- There is no minimum number of measures required. The score will be calculated when the organization meets the case minimum requirement for the two measures, which are:
  — Medicare Spending Per Beneficiary (MSPB)—case minimum = 35 attributed patients
  — Total Per Capita Cost for all attributed beneficiaries—case minimum = 20 attributed patients

Costs are payment standardized, annualized, risk adjusted, and specialty adjusted. Specifically, this means that CMS eliminates the effect of geographic adjustments in payment rates and takes into account risk factors, such as socioeconomic and demographic characteristics, ethnicity, and health status of individuals, in an effort to recognize that less healthy individuals may require more intensive, and thus, more expensive, interventions.

Beginning in 2018, Improvement Scoring will be available for the Cost performance category. The Cost Improvement Score will be calculated by comparing 2018 performance against the 2017 performance and will be reflected in the cost performance category percent score and the 2018 MIPS score. An Improvement bonus of up to one point is available using the net number of measures with improvements versus decline in performance (Figure 3-16).

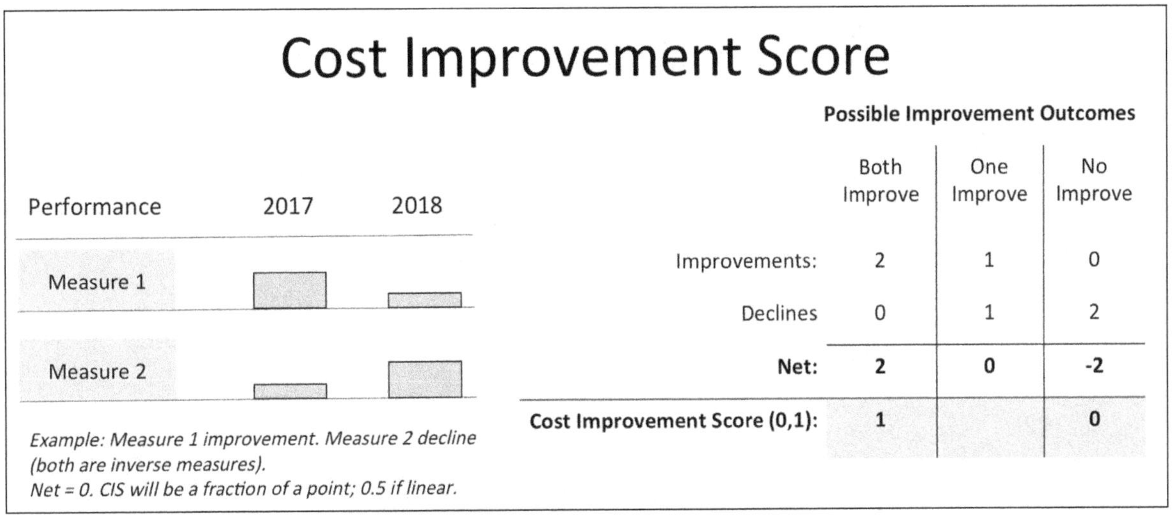

Cost Improvement Score

Possible Improvement Outcomes

Performance	2017	2018		Both Improve	One Improve	No Improve
Measure 1			Improvements:	2	1	0
			Declines	0	1	2
Measure 2			Net:	2	0	-2
			Cost Improvement Score (0,1):	1		0

Example: Measure 1 improvement. Measure 2 decline (both are inverse measures).
Net = 0. CIS will be a fraction of a point; 0.5 if linear.

FIGURE 3-16. Cost Improvement Score

If an individual or group does not receive a Cost score, the weight for the cost category will be redistributed to the Quality category.

Get to Know Your QRUR

The Quality and Resource Use Report (QRUR) is one of the key factors in understanding how many patients are attributed to your TIN and the cost of their care in a calendar year.

QRURs detail aggregate-level data, including information for all NPIs who are associated with the TIN. The QRUR also identifies each of the Medicare beneficiaries that are attributed to a practice and outlines the costs of care associated with them throughout the full continuum of care over the reporting period.

The QRUR will reveal if the costs associated with these patients are at, above, or below national benchmarks. Finding out which patients are attributed to the practice, understanding why they are attributed, and managing that list through several focused initiatives, will be a necessity for scoring well in this category.

QRURs can be accessed through the CMS Enterprise Portal, located at *portal.cms.gov.*

QRURs are how a practice obtains comparative information about the quality and cost of the care provided to Medicare patients. QRURs can be used to:

- Verify the accuracy of Eligible Professionals billing under a groups Tax Identification Number.

If an individual or group does not receive a Cost score, the weight for the cost category will be redistributed to the Quality category.

YOUR TIN'S 2018 VALUE MODIFIER

Average Quality, Average Cost = Neutral Adjustment (0.0%)

Your TIN's overall performance was determined to be average on quality measures and average on cost measures.

This means that the Value Modifier applied to payments for items and services under the Medicare Physician Fee Schedule for clinicians subject to the Value Modifier billing under your TIN in 2018 will result in a neutral adjustment, meaning no adjustment (0.0%).

The scatter plot below shows how your TIN ("You" diamond) compares to a representative sample of other TINs on the Quality and Cost Composite scores used to calculate the 2018 Value Modifier.

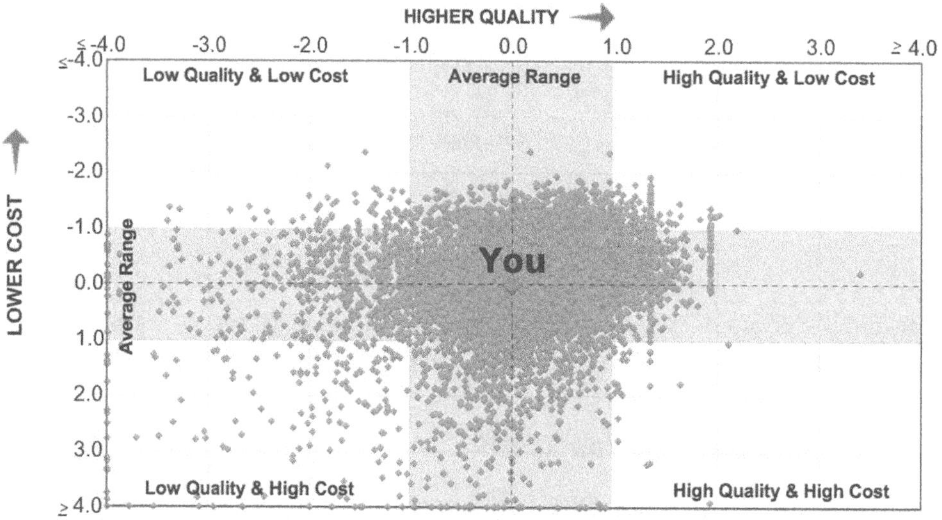

Note: The scatter plot shows performance among a representative sample of all TINs with Quality and Cost Composite Scores reflecting standard deviations from the mean for each Composite Score.

FIGURE 3-17. Your TIN's Value Modifier

- Examine the number of patients attributed to the group as well as the basis for the attribution.
- Evaluate how the group's performance compares to other groups.
- Understand which beneficiaries are driving the group's cost and quality measures.

Below, you'll find screenshots from the cost section of a sample **2016 QRUR** (Remember, this was pre-MIPS, so it used the VM methodology).

The report begins with an illustration showing where the TIN falls in terms of cost and quality performance relative to all other practices as defined by TIN. (See Figure 3-17, Your TIN's Value Modifier.)

Jumping to the Cost section, The Exhibit displays your TIN's Cost Composite Score (the diamond labeled "You") that was used to calculate the VM. The score shows how far your overall performance on cost measures was from the mean for your peer group (with the mean represented as zero).

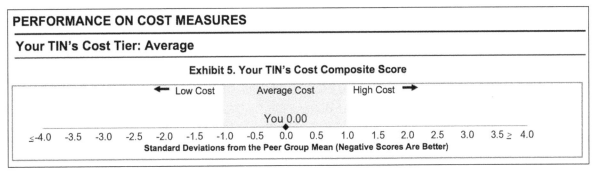

FIGURE 3-18. Performance on Cost Measures

Exhibits 6-A and B. Information Used in the Calculation of Your TIN's Cost Composite Score

A. Summary Cost Performance

Your TIN			All TINs in Peer Group	
Number of Domains Included	Summary Score (Mean Domain Score)	Cost Composite Score (Standardized Summary Score)	Benchmark (Peer Group Mean Summary Score)	Standard Deviation
0	0.00	**0.00**	0.00	0.00

B. Cost Domain Scores

Domain	Number of Measures Included in Domain Score	Domain Score
Costs for All Attributed Beneficiaries	0	0.00
Costs for Beneficiaries with Specific Conditions	0	0.00

FIGURE 3-19. Information Used in the Calculation of Your TIN's Cost Composite Score

The Cost Composite Score standardizes a TIN's cost performance relative to the mean for the TIN's peer group, such that zero represents the peer group mean and the TIN's Cost Composite Score indicates how many standard deviations a TIN's performance is from the mean (Figure 3-18).

Exhibits 6-A and 6-B (Figure 3-19) display a summary of the information used to calculate your TIN's Cost Composite Score. The Cost Composite Score displayed in Exhibit 6- is calculated using the TIN's cost domain scores displayed in Exhibit 6-B. A score for each cost domain is calculated as the equally-weighted average of measure scores within the domain for all measures that have the required minimum number of eligible cases or episodes. Performance is then summarized across all cost domains for which scores could be calculated. This summary score is standardized relative to the mean of summary scores within the TIN's peer group to create the TIN's Cost Composite Score. The Cost Composite Score reflects how many standard deviations from the mean that your TIN's performance across cost domains is. This score is computed by taking the mean of domain scores shown in Exhibit 6-B (also noted as the summary score in Exhibit 6- A), subtracting the benchmark, and dividing the result by the standard deviation displayed in Exhibit 6-A.

All cost measures are classified into two cost domains: the Per Capita Costs for All Attributed Beneficiaries Domain, and the Per Capita Costs for Beneficiaries with Specific Conditions Domain. A score for each cost domain is calculated as the equally weighted average of measure scores within the domain.

In two tables organized by the cost domains detailed above, Exhibit 6 presents 1) your TIN's cost domain scores, and 2) the payment-standard-ized, risk-adjusted, and specialty-adjusted per capita or per episode costs, and the number of eligible cases or episodes for the cost measures.

These measures include the five per capita cost measures (Per Capita Costs for All Attributed Beneficiaries, Per Capita Costs for Beneficiaries with Diabetes, Per Capita Costs for Beneficiaries with COPD, Per Capita Costs for Beneficiaries with CAD, Per Capita Costs for Beneficiaries with Heart Failure) and the MSPB measure that are included in the Value Modifier.

The "Number of Eligible Cases" column in Exhibit 7-AAB displays the number of eligible cases for each measure. The "Standardized Perfor-mance Score" column displays your TIN's score for each measure. The standardized score reflects by how many standard deviations your TIN's performance on a given cost measure differed from the benchmark for that measure. The "Included in Domain Score?" column indicates whether each measure is included in your TIN's domain score. Only the measures for which your TIN met the minimum case size (number of eligible cases or episodes) were included in your TIN's domain score. For the five per capita cost measures, the minimum case size is 20 eligible cases. For the MSPB measure, the minimum case size is 125 eligible cases (Figure 3-20).

Cost data for the Per Capita Costs for All Attributed Beneficiaries measure and the four Per Capita Costs for Beneficiaries with Specific Con-ditions measures are based on Medicare-allowed charges for Medicare Part A and Medicare Part B claims during the period of performance that were submitted by all providers for Medicare beneficiaries attributed to your TIN for these measures. (Exhibit 7-BSC, Figure 3-21). CMS attributes beneficia-ries for these measures to a single TIN through a two-step process that takes into account the level of primary care services received and the provider specialties that performed these services.

With data in hand, you can develop processes to improve performance on cost measures which may involve better data capture, improved com-

Exhibit 7-AAB. Costs for All Attributed Beneficiaries Domain

Domain Score

You 0.00

| ≤-4.0 | -3.0 | -2.0 | -1.0 | 0.0 | 1.0 | 2.0 | 3.0 | ≥ 4.0 |

Standard deviations from the mean domain score (negative scores are better)

	Your TIN				All TINs in Peer Group	
Cost Measure	Number of Eligible Cases or Episodes	Per Capita or Per Episode Costs	Standardized Cost Score	Included in Domain Score?	Benchmark (National Mean)	Standard Deviation
Per Capita Costs for All Attributed Beneficiaries	0	—	0.00	No	$0	$0
Medicare Spending per Beneficiary	0	—	0.00	No	$0	$0

Note: Only the measures for which your TIN had the minimum number of eligible cases or episodes are included in the domain score. For the Per Capita Costs for All Attributed Beneficiaries measure, the minimum number of eligible cases is 20. For the Medicare Spending per Beneficiary measure, the minimum number of eligible episodes is 125. The benchmark for a cost measure is the case-weighted national mean cost among all TINs in the measure's peer group during calendar year 2016. For the Per Capita Costs for All Attributed Beneficiaries measure, the peer group is defined as all TINs nationwide that had at least 20 eligible cases. For the Medicare Spending per Beneficiary measure, the peer group is defined as all TINs nationwide that had at least 125 eligible episodes.

FIGURE 3-20. Costs for All Attributed Beneficiaries

Exhibit 7-BSC. Costs for Beneficiaries with Specific Conditions Domain

Domain Score

You 0.00

| ≤-4.0 | -3.0 | -2.0 | -1.0 | 0.0 | 1.0 | 2.0 | 3.0 | ≥ 4.0 |

Standard deviations from the mean domain score (negative scores are better)

	Your TIN				All TINs in Peer Group	
Cost Measure	Number of Eligible Cases	Per Capita Costs	Standardized Cost Score	Included in Domain Score?	Benchmark (National Mean)	Standard Deviation
Per Capita Costs for Beneficiaries with Diabetes	0	—	0.00	No	$0	$0
Per Capita Costs for Beneficiaries with Chronic Obstructive Pulmonary Disease	0	—	0.00	No	$0	$0
Per Capita Costs for Beneficiaries with Coronary Artery Disease	0	—	0.00	No	$0	$0
Per Capita Costs for Beneficiaries with Heart Failure	0	—	0.00	No	$0	$0

Note: Only the measures for which your TIN had the minimum number of eligible cases are included in the domain score. For the cost measures shown in this exhibit, the minimum number of eligible cases is 20. The benchmark for a cost measure is the case-weighted national mean cost among all TINs in the measure's peer group during calendar year 2016. For the cost measures shown in this exhibit, the peer group is defined as all TINs nationwide that had at least 20 eligible cases for each measure.

FIGURE 3-21. Costs for Beneficiaries with Specific Condit

munication between specialists and primary care, template development, development of protocols of care, assignment of duties to various members of the care team so preventive and other types of care are consistently delivered, all of which tends to result in having lower costs.

Episode-Based Cost Measures Coming in Future Years

CMS is in the process of developing and field-testing eight episode-based cost measures to include in MIPS in future years along with extensive feedback from clinicians in the industry. Although these are not included in the 2018 performance year, understanding CMS's methodology can feel overwhelming, so it's worth the effort to start wrapping your head around the topic sooner rather than later.

CMS has been seeking stakeholder feedback in the development of cost measures for several years now and they are incorporating what they've learned so far. Their key findings have been:

- Defining episode groups and cost measures must yield actionable information that can guide improvements to patient care.
- Assignment of costs to episode groups should only hold clinicians accountable for patient outcomes that are within the scope implied by their clinical role.
- Attribution of claims and episodes to clinicians should be clear and credible at the time of service.
- Cost measures should account for patient complexity through appropriate risk adjustment.
- Cost measures must be aligned with quality measures.
- Broad stakeholder feedback is crucial to the development and implementation process.

The eight episode-based cost measures being developed include:
1. Elective Outpatient Percutaneous Coronary Intervention (PCI)
2. Knee Arthroplasty
3. Revascularization for Lower Extremity Chronic Critical Limp Ischemia
4. Routine Cataract Removal with Intraocular Lens (IOL) Implantation
5. Screening/Surveillance Colonoscopy
6. Intracranial Hemorrhage or Cerebral Infarction
7. Simple Pneumonia with Hospitalization
8. ST-Elevation Myocardial Infarction (STEMI) with PCI

Episode-based cost measures represent the cost to Medicare for the items and services furnished to a patient during an episode of care. They are being developed to let clinicians know the cost of care they are responsible for providing to a beneficiary during an episode's timeframe.

A cost measure has five essential components:

1. Defining the Episode Group
2. Attributing the Episode Group to Clinicians
3. Assigning Costs to the Episode Group
4. Risk Adjusting Episode Groups
5. Aligning Cost with Quality

Let's take a moment to dig deeper into each component.

1. Defining the Episode Group

   - *An episode group focuses on clinical conditions requiring treatment (the condition itself or procedures to treat the condition)*
     — Example: A procedural episode group that is surgical in nature could include: pre-operative services, surgical procedure, anesthesia, follow-up care, services related to complications, and readmissions
   - *An episode is a specific instance of an episode group for a given patient and clinician*
     — Example: A clinician might be attributed 20 episodes (instances of the episode group) from the knee arthroplasty episode group in a year.
   - *Can vary in scope (e.g. narrow and precise or broad and general)*
     — Example: An episode group for cataract removal with insertion of intraocular lens prosthesis has a narrow scope. In comparison, an episode group for gastrointestinal hemorrhage has a broad scope.
   - *Can be divided into sub-groups to define more homogenous patient cohorts*
     — Example: Gastrointestinal hemorrhage may be divided into sub-groups for upper and lower gastrointestinal hemorrhage.
   - *There are three types of Episode Groups:*
     — *Acute Inpatient Medical Condition* episode groups represent treatment for self-limited acute illness or treatment for flares or an exacerbation of a condition that requires a hospital stay. Of the eight measures in field testing, three are based on acute inpatient medical condition episode groups: Intracranial Hemorrhage or Cerebral Infarction, Simple Pneumonia with Hospitalization, and STEMI with PCI.
     — *Chronic Condition* episode groups account for the patient's clinical history at the time of a medical visit and their current health status. An example of a chronic condition episode group is an episode group for the ongoing management of a disease, such as diabetes.
     — *Procedural* episode groups focus on procedures of a defined purpose or type, such as surgeries. Of the eight measures in field testing, five are based on procedural episode groups: Elective Outpatient PCI, Knee Arthroplasty, Revascularization for Lower Extremity

Chronic Critical Limb Ischemia, Routine Cataract Removal with IOL Implantation, and Screening/Surveillance Colonoscopy.

2. Attributing the Episode Group to Clinicians
   - Attribution is the assignment of responsibility for an episode of care to a principal (or managing) clinician based on the trigger event.
   - Attribution should be transparent to clinicians and only hold them responsible for outcomes they can reasonably be expected to influence.
   - Patient relationship categories and codes that are being developed under MACRA can be evaluated in the future to determine how they could potentially be used with claims-based measures.

3. Assigning Costs to the Episode Group
   - Assignment of items and services determines what is included in episode costs and depends on role of the attributed clinician.
   - Episode window determines the period of time during which claims are eligible to be assigned to the episode.

   Items and Services that *are* assigned to the Episode Group:
   - Treatment services
   - Diagnostic services
   - Ancillary care directly related to treatment (e.g., anesthesia for a surgical procedure)
   - Consequences of care (e.g., complications, readmissions, unplanned care, emergency department visits)

   Items and Services that *are not* assigned to the Episode Group:
   - Unrelated Services—unrelated to the clinical management of the patient's condition or procedure that is the focus of the episode group

4. Risk Adjusting Episode Groups
   - Adjust for factors outside the clinician's control that can influence spending.
     — i.e. age, illness severity, comorbidities, other aspects of patient's clinical history
   - Aim to isolate the variation in clinician's costs to Medicare to those costs clinicians can reasonably control.
   - Accounting for these factors is one way to ensure the validity of the measures and mitigate potential unintended consequences.
   - Select risk adjustment method informed by empirical analyses, technical expert panels, clinical subcommittees, and public comment.

5. Aligning Cost with Quality
   - Alignment with indicators of quality is necessary to ensure that clinicians throughout a patient's care trajectory are incentivized to provide high-value, patient-centered care
   - Quality assessments might include:

- Complications, re-hospitalizations, unplanned care, and other consequences
- Outcomes of care
- Overuse, underuse, misuse of orders, tests, imaging, etc.
- Processes of care
- Functional status of patient
- Patient experience

Hierarchical Condition Categories (HCC) and Risk Adjustment Factor's (RAF) Role

Under MIPS, clinical documentation and coding specificity can have a big impact. Medicare patients have a default risk adjustment factor (RAF) based on their demographics, that when combined with their Hierarchical Condition Categories (HCC) and diagnosis codes for chronic conditions will modify their RAF score. By being more specific about the severity and complexity of the condition, the patient's risk score can increase substantially.

More specific coding allows payments to be risk-adjusted based on patient complexity. Since the allowable costs are contingent upon the risk scores of the patient population attributed to the practice, if you are not specific in your coding, it will be difficult to demonstrate that you can care for complex patients in a low cost manner. Accurate coding information helps create a more complete picture of a patient population's complexity, and enables better management of a patient's chronic diseases.

HCC is the basis for CMS to determine your risk adjustment and how you code your claims will determine the HCC for your patients. Thankfully, you're not limited to four diagnoses per claim any longer—you can submit up to 12 in an electronic claim.

At its core, diagnosis codes (ICD-10) are assigned a weight that measures patient acuity. CMS has experienced, as a general rule, that patients with higher HCC scores will consume more healthcare dollars and have worse outcomes.

Using more specific ICD-10 coding can impact the risk adjustment factor (RAF) of your patient mix, which could contribute to qualifying for a complex patient bonus of up to five points, a process described in the "Calculating the Composite Score" section (Table 3-25).

Internal expertise and communication among coding and documentation staff will be paramount to coding success as practices advance with QPP plans. Practice coders who extract data for claims from clinical documentation can only code what is available in the patient chart or encounter note. Thus, physician education on coding requirements is vital. Documen-

Thus, physician education on coding requirements is vital. Documentation by physicians must be thorough and granular enough to support the right degree of acuity in claims reporting.

TABLE 3-25. How Coding More Specifically Affects the Risk Adjustment Factor

Non-Specific Coding		Specific Coding	
ICD 10 Code	RAF	ICD 10 Code	RAF
Demographic RAF*	0.390	Demographic RAF*	0.390
E11.9 Type II diabetes mellitus without complications	0.104	E11.22 Type II diabetes mellitus with diabetic chronic kidney disease	0.318
N18.9 Chronic kidney disease, unspecified	0.000	N18.4 Chronic kidney disease, stage 4	0.237
E66.9 Obesity unspecified	0.000	E66.01 Morbid obesity	0.273
F32.8 Other depressive episodes	0.000	F32.1 Major depressive illness, single episode, moderately severe	0.395
I25.9 Chronic ischemic heart disease, unspecified	0.000	I25.119 Atherosclerotic heart disease of native coronary artery with unspecified angina pectoris	0.140
Total**	0.494	Total**	1.753

* Average demographic Risk Adjustment Factor (RAF), 2016
** Average RAF for FFS Medicare patient: 1.0

tation by physicians must be thorough and granular enough to support the right degree of acuity in claims reporting.

In practices where clinicians are coding for themselves, the onus is on physicians to stay abreast of coding guidelines and protocols. Physicians using electronic health record (EHR) dropdowns for coding may benefit from training on how to quickly and effectively find diagnostic terms in the alphabetical index, which can be challenging for reasons related to classification labeling specifics. Establishing familiarity with ICD-10 codes most commonly used in a practice is the best place to start.

Keys to Success

The calculation of the two Cost measures requires data that is not easily available to most practices. This, combined with the same year benchmark methodology, makes it difficult to plan ahead. However, there are several strategies you can use to get ready:

- Building the right infrastructure now will yield results in the future.
- Remember that levers for success depend on the environment in which you are practicing.
- Designate a person to access QRUR and Feedback reports through the EIDM portal.

- Review your prior year QRURs to understand your historical cost performance.
- Know which patients are attributed to your practice.
- Target, track, and treat high-risk patients identified in QRUR.
- Target areas of high-cost in QRUR.
- Provide dedicated time to work on improvement.
- Design workflows for population management.
- Run lists of patients by diagnosis and identify care gaps.
- Consider making an additional spreadsheet.
- Where are areas for easy improvement?
  — Compare trouble areas with selected quality measures—is there alignment?
- Where are areas for long-term improvement?
  — Compare trouble areas with Improvement Activities.
- Population health
  — Prevention/screenings
  — Registries—disease management
  — Addressing unique characteristics of geographic area
- Follow-up with discharge patients
  — Billable services (Transitional Care Management)
  — Reduction in ambulatory care-sensitive conditions
  — Management of chronic conditions (CCM)
  — Patient engagement
  — Improve patient satisfaction/compliance
- Analyze your 2017 cost performance category score as soon as it becomes available. Remember, this score would be used as the basis for calculating improvement of your 2018 cost category performance score.
- Keep in mind that performance will be influenced not only by the charges originating from the group of providers being evaluated, but also by other providers who see the same patients.
- Keep patients coming back to your practice.
- Have a referral network in place with providers who share your approach and who are mindful of controlling cost and providing good care.
- Establish transitions of care process with hospitals, home health, skilled nursing facilities, and specialists.
- Have coders study measure specifications to ensure reporting is accurate and specific; code robustly!

Resources

- https://www.cms.gov/Medicare/Quality-Payment-Program/Resource-Library/2018-Resources.html

- How to Obtain a QRUR: https://www.cms.gov/Medicare/Medicare-Fee-for-Service-Payment/PhysicianFeedbackProgram/Downloads/2016-QRUR-Guide.pdf
- Understanding Your QRUR: https://www.cms.gov/Medicare/Medicare-Fee-for-Service-Payment/PhysicianFeedbackProgram/Downloads/2016-UnderstandingYourAQRUR.pdf
- Measure Information about the Medicare Spending Per Beneficiary: https://www.cms.gov/Medicare/Medicare-Fee-for-Service-Payment/PhysicianFeedbackProgram/Downloads/2016-MSPBM-MIF.pdf
- Measure Information about the Total Per Capita Costs Measure: https://www.cms.gov/Medicare/Medicare-Fee-for-Service-Payment/PhysicianFeedbackProgram/Downloads/2016-TPCC-MIF.pdf
- Episode-Based Cost Measure Field Test Reports Fact Sheet: https://www.cms.gov/Medicare/Quality-Initiatives-Patient-Assessment-Instruments/Value-Based-Programs/MACRA-MIPS-and-APMs/Cost-Measures-Field-Test-Fact-Sheet.pdf
- CMS Risk Adjustment Fact Sheet: https://www.cms.gov/Medicare/Medicare-Fee-for-Service-Payment/PhysicianFeedbackProgram/Downloads/2015-RiskAdj-FactSheet.pdf

Lessons Learned from the Field

Lesson 1: Know your attributed patients.

The dollars that your attributed patients spend throughout the healthcare system over the course of a year can essentially be translated to *your* costs. This means that if you have a large portion of patients with diabetes that goes untreated until until eventual hospitalization, the cost to the healthcare system on a whole is greater than it would be had these patients taken a more proactive approach. In other words, a little preventive maintenance, in theory, should eliminate the need for major repairs.

The importance cannot be stressed enough: know which patients (and their associated costs) are attributed to you. You may find a subset of them that don't have a primary care physician, but should, or that have not sought treatment for their high-risk conditions, or who were hospitalized for something that could have been prevented and/or requires follow-up care upon discharge.

Your goal should not be to have as few patients on your attribution list as possible. Instead, it should be to ensure that the patients who are attributed to you are on your list for the right reasons. Once that is established, do your best to make sure those patients are taking a proactive approach to maintaining their health.

Lesson 2: Get better at coordinating care.

Once you know your patients and identify the ones with high-risk conditions, then you can start building your referral network to meet those patients' needs. If you have a high population of attributed patients with a specific diagnosis of heart failure, COPD, coronary artery disease, or diabetes, start connecting with specialists who treat their primary ailments and common symptoms. Your network might include practices with the following concentration:

- Primary Care
- Cardiology
- Endocrinology
- Pulmonology
- Urology
- Podiatry
- Gastroenterology
- Oncology
- Dermatology
- Respiratory therapy
- Dietician/nutritionist
- Exercise specialist
- Therapist or counselor

Considering the overarching goals of the QPP, theoretically the patient's heath data should be able to follow her to any doctor's office of her choosing. One of the most efficient and, more importantly, secure ways of sharing this highly sensitive data is to utilize the Direct Mail feature, typically accessed through the internal/external mailbox of your EHR. Direct Mail is inherently a HIPAA-secure email that is capable of safely sending and receiving encrypted files that contain electronic Protected Health Information (ePHI). It is quickly becoming the industry standard for sharing patient records and "closing the referral loop."

If you haven't started leveraging the capabilities of your EHR in this way yet, well, what are you waiting for?

If you're a dermatologist and you happen to have a high number of attributed patients with diabetes, for example, it doesn't mean you now need to start treating diabetes. What it means is that your professional recommendation that they follow-up with their primary care physician or other healthcare professional is likely to result in their following your directions. Over time, the hope for and intended results of this approach is for healthier patient outcomes.

It's like that saying: a pound of prevention is worth an ounce of cure.

Lesson 3: Know the hospitals in your network.

One of the most expensive items that can negatively impact your cost metrics is when one of your attributed patients has a hospital stay.

For each hospital visit, CMS tracks the patient's admission date, principal diagnosis, and length of stay.

Similar to the Physician Compare website, CMS has a Hospital Compare website, where they publish star ratings based on summarizing 57 quality measures reflecting common conditions that hospitals treat, such as heart attacks or pneumonia. The overall rating shows how well each hospital performed, on average, compared to other hospitals in the U.S.

In an emergency, obviously, patients should go to the nearest hospital. However, when patients are able to plan ahead, the Hospital Compare overall rating can provide a starting point for comparing a hospital to others locally, regionally, and nationwide.

If possible, work toward building a relationship with the hospitals in your community so you can be advised when your attributed patients are admitted, discharged, and/or require follow-up care.

IMPROVEMENT ACTIVITIES

The improvement activities performance category focuses on one of CMS' MIPS strategic goals, to use a patient-centered approach to program development that leads to better, smarter, and healthier care. CMS believes improving the health of all Americans can be accomplished by developing incentives and policies that drive improved patient health outcomes. Improvement activities emphasize actions that have a proven association with better health outcomes.

This category was brand new for every clinician as of 2017 and it consists of participating in activities with one of the following themes:

- Expand Practice Access
- Population Management
- Care Coordination
- Beneficiary Engagement
- Patient Safety and Practice Assessment
- Achieving Health Equity
- Integrated Behavioral and Mental Health

CMS has identified more than 100 activities that can be used for earning points in this category. Improvement Activities can be anything from communicating test results in a timely manner, using decision support and protocols to manage workflows, providing self-management materials to patients, to offering them 24/7 access to urgent and emergent care.

Some activities carry more weight than others and providers must demonstrate that the activity has happened for at least 90 days to get credit (Figure 3-22, Table 3-26).

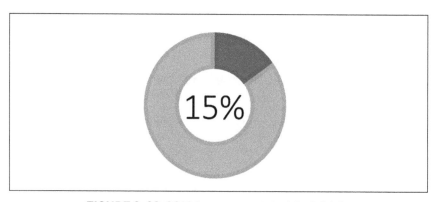

FIGURE 3-22. 2018 Improvement Activity Weight

List of Improvement Activities (Table 3-26)

TABLE 3-26. List of Improvement Activities

Subcategory	Activity Title + Description	Weight	Activity ID
Expanded Practice Access	Provide 24/7 Access to MIPS-eligible Clinicians or Groups Who Have Real- Time Access to Patient's Medical Record Provide 24/7 access to MIPS-eligible clinicians, groups, or care teams for advice about urgent and emergent care (e.g., MIPS-eligible clinician and care team access to medical record, cross-coverage with access to medical record, or protocol-driven nurse line with access to medical record) that could include one or more of the following: • Expanded hours in evenings and weekends with access to the patient medical record (e.g., coordinate with small practices to provide alternate hour office visits and urgent care); • Use of alternatives to increase access to care team by MIPS-eligible clinicians and groups, such as e-visits, phone visits, group visits, home visits and alternate locations (e.g., senior centers and assisted living centers); and/or • Provision of same-day or next-day access to a consistent MIPS-eligible clinician, group, or care team, when needed for urgent care or transition management.	High	IA_EPA_1
Expanded Practice Access	Use of Telehealth Services that Expand Practice Access Use of telehealth services and analysis of data for quality improvement, such as participation in remote specialty care consults, or teleaudiology pilots that assess ability to still deliver quality care to patients.	Medium	IA_EPA_2
Expanded Practice Access	Collection and Use of Patient Experience and Satisfaction Data on Access Collection of patient experience and satisfaction data on access to care and development of an improvement plan, such as outlining steps for improving communications with patients to help understanding of urgent access needs.	Medium	IA_EPA_3
Expanded Practice Access	Additional Improvements in Access as a Result of QIN/QIO TA As a result of Quality Innovation Network-Quality Improvement Organization technical assistance, performance of additional activities that improve access to services (e.g., investment of on-site diabetes educator).	Medium	IA_EPA_4
Population Management	Participation in a Systematic Anticoagulation Program Participation in a systematic anticoagulation program (coagulation clinic, patient self-reporting program, or patient self-management program) for 60 percent of practice patients in the transition year and 75 percent of practice patients in Quality Payment Program Year 2 and future years, who receive anti-coagulation medications (warfarin or other coagulation cascade inhibitors).	High	IA_PM_1

(continued on next page)

TABLE 3-26. List of Improvement Activities (continued)

Subcategory	Activity Title + Description	Weight	Activity ID
Population Management	**Anticoagulant Management Improvements** Individual MIPS-eligible clinicians and groups who prescribe oral Vitamin K antagonist therapy (warfarin) must attest that, for 60 percent of practice patients in the transition year and 75 percent of practice patients in Quality Payment Program Year 2 and future years, their ambulatory care patients receiving warfarin are being managed by one or more of the following improvement activities: • Patients are being managed by an anticoagulant management service, that involves systematic and coordinated care, incorporating comprehensive patient education, systematic prothrombin time (PT- INR) testing, tracking, follow-up, and patient communication of results and dosing decisions; • Patients are being managed according to validated electronic decision support and clinical management tools that involve systematic and coordinated care, incorporating comprehensive patient education, systematic PT-INR testing, tracking, follow-up, and patient communication of results and dosing decisions; • For rural or remote patients, patients are managed using remote monitoring or telehealth options that involve systematic and coordinated care, incorporating comprehensive patient education, systematic PT-INR testing, tracking, follow-up, and patient communication of results and dosing decisions; and/or • For patients who demonstrate motivation, competency, and adherence, patients are managed using either a patient self-testing (PST) or patient-self-management (PSM) program.	High	IA_PM_2
Population Management	**RHC, HIS, or FQHC Quality Improvement Activities** Participating in a Rural Health Clinic (RHC), Indian Health Service (IHS), or Federally Qualified Health Center in ongoing engagement activities that contribute to more formal quality reporting, and that include receiving quality data back for broader quality improvement and benchmarking improvement which will ultimately benefit patients. Participation in Indian Health Service, as an improvement activity, requires MIPS-eligible clinicians and groups to deliver care to federally recognized American Indian and Alaska Native populations in the U.S. and in the course of that care, implement continuous clinical practice improvement including reporting data on quality of services being provided and receiving feedback to make improvements over time.	High	IA_PM_3
Population Management	**Glycemic Management Services** For outpatient Medicare beneficiaries with diabetes and who are prescribed antidiabetic agents (e.g., insulin, sulfonylureas), MIPS-eligible clinicians and groups must attest to having: For the first performance year, at least 60 percent of medical records with documentation of an individualized glycemic treatment goal that: a. Takes into account patient-specific factors, including, at least 1) age, 2) comorbidities, and 3) risk for hypoglycemia, and b. Is reassessed at least annually. The performance threshold will increase to 75 percent for the second performance year and onward. Clinicians would attest that 60 percent for the transition year or 75 percent for the second year of their medical records document individualized glycemic treatment represent patients who are being treated for at least 90 days during the performance period.	High	IA_PM_4

(continued on next page)

TABLE 3-26. List of Improvement Activities (continued)

Subcategory	Activity Title + Description	Weight	Activity ID
Population Management	Engagement of Community for Health Status Improvement Take steps to improve health status of communities, such as collaborating with key partners and stakeholders to implement evidenced-based practices to improve a specific chronic condition. Refer to the local Quality Improvement Organization (QIO) for additional steps to take for improving health status of communities as there are many steps to select from for satisfying this activity. QIOs work under the direction of CMS to assist MIPS-eligible clinicians and groups with quality improvement, and review quality concerns for the protection of beneficiaries and the Medicare Trust Fund.	Medium	IA_PM_5
Population Management	Use of Toolsets or Other Resources to Close Healthcare Disparities across Communities Take steps to improve healthcare disparities, such as use of Population Health Toolkit or other resources identified by CMS, the Learning and Action Network, Quality Innovation Network, or National Coordinating Center. Refer to the local Quality Improvement Organization (QIO) for additional steps to take for improving health status of communities, as there are many steps to select from for satisfying this activity. QIOs work under the direction of CMS to assist eligible clinicians and groups with quality improvement and review quality concerns for the protection of beneficiaries and the Medicare Trust Fund.	Medium	IA_PM_6
Population Management	Use of a QCDR for Feedback Reports that Incorporate Population Health Use of a QCDR to generate regular feedback reports that summarize local practice patterns and treatment outcomes, including for vulnerable populations.	High	IA_PM_7
Population Management	Participation in Population Health Research Participation in research that identifies interventions, tools, or processes that can improve a targeted patient population.	Medium	IA_PM_9
Population Management	Use of QCDR Data for Quality Improvements such as Comparative Analysis Reports across Patient Populations Participation in a QCDR, clinical data registries, or other registries run by other government agencies such as FDA, or private entities such as a hospital or medical or surgical society. Activity must include use of QCDR data for quality improvement (e.g., comparative analysis across specific patient populations for adverse outcomes after an outpatient surgical procedure and corrective steps to address adverse outcome).	Medium	IA_PM_10
Population Management	Regular Review Practices in Place on Targeted Patient Population Needs Implementation of regular reviews of targeted patient population needs, such as structured clinical case reviews, which includes access to reports that show unique characteristics of eligible clinician's patient population, identification of vulnerable patients, and how clinical treatment needs are being tailored, if necessary, to address unique needs and what resources in the community have been identified as additional resources.	Medium	IA_PM_11

(continued on next page)

TABLE 3-26. List of Improvement Activities (continued)

Subcategory	Activity Title + Description	Weight	Activity ID
Population Management	**Population Empanelment** Empanel (assign responsibility for) the total population, linking each patient to an MIPS-eligible clinician or group or care team. Empanelment is a series of processes that assign each active patient to an MIPS-eligible clinician or group and/or care team, confirm assignment with patients and clinicians, and use the resultant patient panels as a foundation for individual patient and population health management. Empanelment identifies the patients and population for whom the MIPS-eligible clinician or group and/or care team is responsible and is the foundation for the relationship continuity between patient and MIPS-eligible clinician or group /care team that is at the heart of comprehensive primary care. Effective empanelment requires identification of the "active population" of the practice: those patients who identify and use your practice as a source for primary care. There are many ways to define "active patients" operationally, but generally, the definition of "active patients" includes patients who have sought care within the last 24 to 36 months, allowing inclusion of younger patients who have minimal acute or preventive health care.	Medium	IA_PM_12
Population Management	**Chronic Care and Preventative Care Management for Empaneled Patients** Proactively manage chronic and preventive care for empaneled patients that could include one or more of the following: Provide patients annually with an opportunity for development and/or adjustment of an individualized plan of care as appropriate to age and health status, including health risk appraisal (gender, age and condition-specific preventive care services), and plan of care for chronic conditions; • Use condition-specific pathways for care of chronic conditions (e.g., hypertension, diabetes, depression, asthma and heart failure) with evidence-based protocols to guide treatment to target, such as a CDC- recognized diabetes prevention program; • Use pre-visit planning to optimize preventive care and team management of patients with chronic conditions; • Use panel support tools (registry functionality) to identify services due; • Use predictive analytical models to predict risk, onset, and progression of chronic diseases; or • Use reminders and outreach (e.g., phone calls, emails, postcards, patient portals, and community health workers where available) to alert and educate patients about services due, and/or routine medication reconciliation.	Medium	IA_PM_13
Population Management	**Implementation of Methodologies for Improvements in Longitudinal Care Management for High Risk Patients** Provide longitudinal care management to patients at high risk for adverse health outcomes or harm that could include one or more of the following: • Use a consistent method to assign and adjust global risk status for all empaneled patients to allow risk stratification into actionable risk cohorts. Monitor the risk-stratification method and refine as necessary to improve accuracy of risk status identification; • Use a personalized plan of care for patients at high risk for adverse health outcome or harm, integrating patient goals, values, and priorities; and/or • Use on-site practice-based or shared care managers to proactively monitor and coordinate care for the highest risk cohort of patients.	Medium	IA_PM_14

(continued on next page)

TABLE 3-26. List of Improvement Activities (continued)

Subcategory	Activity Title + Description	Weight	Activity ID
Population Management	Implementation of Episodic Care Management Practice Improvements Provide episodic care management, including management across transitions and referrals that could include one or more of the following: • Routine and timely follow-up to hospitalizations, ED visits and stays in other institutional settings, including symptom and disease management, and medication reconciliation and management; and/or • Managing care intensively through new diagnoses, injuries and exacerbations of illness.	Medium	IA_PM_15
Population Management	Implementation of Medication Management Practice Improvements Manage medications to maximize efficiency, effectiveness, and safety that could include one or more of the following: • Reconcile and coordinate medications and provide medication management across transitions of care settings and eligible clinicians or groups; • Integrate a pharmacist into the care team; and/or Conduct periodic, structured medication reviews.	Medium	IA_PM_16
Population Management	Participation in Population Health Research Participation in federally and/or privately funded research that identifies interventions, tools, or processes that can improve a targeted patient population.	Medium	IA_PM_17
Population Management	Provide Clinical-Community Linkages Engage community health workers to provide a comprehensive link to community resources through family-based services focusing on success in health, education, and self-sufficiency. This activity supports individual MIPS-eligible clinicians or groups that coordinate with primary care and other clinicians, engage and support patients, use health information technology, and employ quality measurement and improvement processes. An example of this community-based program is the NCQA Patient-Centered Connected Care (PCCC) Recognition Program or other such programs that meet these criteria.	Medium	IA_PM_18
Population Management	Glycemic Screening Services For at-risk outpatient Medicare beneficiaries, individual MIPS-eligible clinicians and groups must attest to implementation of systematic preventive approaches in clinical practice, for at least 60 percent for the 2018 performance period and 75 percent in future years, of electronic medical records with documentation of screening patients for abnormal blood glucose in accordance with current US Preventive Services Task Force (USPSTF) and/or American Diabetes Association (ADA) guidelines.	Medium	IA_PM_19
Population Management	Glycemic Referring Services For at-risk outpatient Medicare beneficiaries, individual MIPS-eligible clinicians and groups must attest to implementation of systematic preventive approaches in clinical practice, for at least 60 percent for the CY 2018 performance period and 75 percent in future years, of medical records with documentation of referring eligible patients with pre-diabetes to a CDC-recognized diabetes prevention program operating under the framework of the National Diabetes Prevention Program.	Medium	IA_PM_20

(continued on next page)

TABLE 3-26. List of Improvement Activities (continued)

Subcategory	Activity Title + Description	Weight	Activity ID
Population Management	Advance Care Planning Implement practices/processes to develop advance care planning that include: documenting the advance care plan or living will within the medical record, educating clinicians about advance care planning and motivating them to address the advance care planning needs of their patients, as well as how these needs can translate into quality improvement. Educate clinicians on approaches and barriers to talking to patients about end-of-life and palliative care needs and ways to manage their documentation, as well as inform clinicians of the healthcare policy side of advance care planning.	Medium	IA_PM_21
Care Coordination	Implementation of Use of Specialist Reports Back to Referring Clinician or Group to Close Referral Loop Performance of regular practices that include providing specialist reports back to the referring individual MIPS-eligible clinician or group to close the referral loop or where the referring individual MIPS-eligible clinician, or group initiates regular inquiries to specialists for specialist reports which could be documented or noted in the EHR technology.	Medium	IA_CC_1
Care Coordination	Implementation of Improvements that Contribute to More Timely Communication of Test Results Timely communication of test results are defined as timely identification of abnormal test results with timely follow-up.	Medium	IA_CC_2
Care Coordination	Implementation of Additional Activity as a Result of TA for Improving Care Coordination Implementation of at least one additional recommended activity from the Quality Innovation Network-Quality Improvement Organization after technical assistance has been provided related to improving care coordination.	Medium	IA_CC_3
Care Coordination	TCPI Participation Participation in the CMS Transforming Clinical Practice Initiative (TCPI).	Medium	IA_CC_4
Care Coordination	CMS Partner in Patients Hospital Improvement Innovations Network Membership and participation in a CMS Partnership for Patients Hospital Improvement Innovation Network.	Medium	IA_CC_5
Care Coordination	Use of QCDR to Promote Standard Practices, Tools and Processes in Practice for Improvement in Care Coordination Participation in a Qualified Clinical Data Registry, demonstrating performance of activities that promote use of standard practices, tools, and processes for quality improvement (e.g., documented preventative screening and vaccinations that can be shared across MIPS-eligible clinician or groups).	Medium	IA_CC_6
Care Coordination	Regular Training in Care Coordination Implementation of regular care coordination training.	Medium	IA_CC_7
Care Coordination	Implementation of Documentation Improvements for Practice/Process Improvements Implementation of practices/processes that document care coordination activities (e.g., a documented care coordination encounter that tracks all clinical staff involved and communications from date patient is scheduled for outpatient procedure through day of procedure).	Medium	IA_CC_8

(continued on next page)

TABLE 3-26. List of Improvement Activities (continued)

Subcategory	Activity Title + Description	Weight	Activity ID
Care Coordination	Implementation of Practices/Processes for Developing Regular Individual Care Plans. Implementation of practices/processes, including a discussion on care, to develop regularly updated individual care plans for at-risk patients that are shared with the beneficiary or caregiver(s). Individual care plans should include consideration of a patient's goals and priorities, as well as desired outcomes of care.	Medium	IA_CC_9
Care Coordination	Care Transition Documentation Practice Improvements Implementation of practices/processes for care transition that include documentation of how a MIPS-eligible clinician or group carried out a patient-centered action plan for the first 30 days following a discharge (e.g., staff involvement, phone calls conducted in support of transition, accompaniments, navigation actions, home visits, patient information access, etc.).	Medium	IA_CC_10
Care Coordination	Care Transition Standard Operational Improvements Establish standard operations to manage transitions of care that could include one or more of the following: • Establish formalized lines of communication with local settings in which empaneled patients receive care to ensure documented flow of information and seamless transitions in care; and/or • Partner with community or hospital-based transitional care services.	Medium	IA_CC_11
Care Coordination	Care Coordination Agreements that Promote Improvements in Patient Tracking across Settings Establish effective care coordination and active referral management that could include one or more of the following: 1. Establish care coordination agreements with frequently used consultants that set expectations for documented flow of information and MIPS-eligible clinician or MIPS-eligible clinician group expectations between settings. Provide patients with information that consistently sets their expectations with the care coordination agreements; 2. Track patients referred to a specialist through the entire process; and/or 3. Systematically integrate information from referrals into the plan of care.	Medium	IA_CC_12
Care Coordination	Practice Improvements for Bilateral Exchange of Patient Information Ensure that there is bilateral exchange of necessary patient information to guide patient care, such as Open Notes, that could include one or more of the following: • Participate in a Health Information Exchange if available; and/or • Use structured referral notes.	Medium	IA_CC_13

(continued on next page)

TABLE 3-26. List of Improvement Activities (continued)

Subcategory	Activity Title + Description	Weight	Activity ID
Care Coordination	**Practice Improvements that Engage Community Resources to Support Patient Health Goals** Develop pathways to neighborhood/community-based resources to support patient health goals that could include one or more of the following: • Maintain formal (referral) links to community-based chronic disease self-management support programs, exercise programs, and other wellness resources with the potential for bidirectional flow of information; and provide a guide to available community resources, including through the use of tools that facilitate electronic communication between settings; • Screen patients for health-harming legal needs; • Screen and assess patients for social needs using tools that are preferably health IT enabled and that include, to any extent, standards-based, coded question/field for the capture of data as is feasible and available as part of such tool; and/or • Provide a guide to available community resources.	Medium	IA_CC_14
Care Coordination	**Perioperative Surgical Home (PSH) Care Coordination** Participate in a Perioperative Surgical Home (PSH) that provides a patient-centered, physician-led, interdisciplinary, and team-based system of coordinated patient care, which coordinates care from pre-procedure assessment through the acute care episode, recovery, and post-acute care. This activity allows for reporting of strategies and processes related to care coordination of patients receiving surgical or procedural care within a PSH. The clinician must perform one or more of the following care coordination activities: • Coordinate with care managers/navigators in preoperative clinic to plan and implement comprehensive post discharge plan of care; • Deploy perioperative clinic and care processes to reduce post-operative visits to emergency rooms; • Implement evidence-informed practices and standardize care across the entire spectrum of surgical patients; or • Implement processes to ensure effective communications and education of patients' post-discharge instructions.	Medium	IA_CC_15
Care Coordination	**Primary Care Physician and Behavioral Health Bilateral Electronic Exchange of Information for Shared Patients** The primary care and behavioral health practices use the same electronic health record system for shared patients or have an established bidirectional flow of primary care and behavioral health records.	Medium	IA_CC_16
Care Coordination	**Patient Navigator Program** Implement a Patient Navigator Program that offers evidence-based resources and tools to reduce avoidable hospital readmissions, utilizing a patient-centered and team-based approach, and leveraging evidence-based best practices to improve care for patients by making hospitalizations less stressful and making the recovery period more supportive by implementing quality improvement strategies.	High	IA_CC_17
Beneficiary Engagement	**Use of Certified EHR to Capture Patient Reported Outcomes** In support of improving patient access, performing additional activities that enable capture of patient reported outcomes (e.g., home blood pressure, blood glucose logs, food diaries, at-risk health factors such as tobacco or alcohol use, etc.) or patient activation measures through use of certified EHR technology, and contain this data in a separate queue for clinician recognition and review.	Medium	IA_BE_1

(continued on next page)

TABLE 3-26. List of Improvement Activities (continued)

Subcategory	Activity Title + Description	Weight	Activity ID
Beneficiary Engagement	Use of QCDR to Support Clinical Decision Making Participation in a QCDR, demonstrating performance of activities that promote implementation of shared clinical decision making capabilities.	Medium	IA_BE_2
Beneficiary Engagement	Engagement with QIN-QIO to Implement Self-Management Training Programs Engagement with a Quality Innovation Network-Quality Improvement Organization, which may include participation in self-management training programs such as diabetes.	Medium	IA_BE_3
Beneficiary Engagement	Engagement of Patients through Implementation of Improvements in Patient Portal Access to an enhanced patient portal that provides up to date information related to relevant chronic disease health or blood pressure control, and includes interactive features allowing patients to enter health information and/or enables bidirectional communication about medication changes and adherence.	Medium	IA_BE_4
Beneficiary Engagement	Enhancements/Regular Updates to Practice Websites/Tools that Also Include Considerations for Patients with Cognitive Disabilities Enhancements and ongoing regular updates and use of websites/tools that include consideration for compliance with section 508 of the Rehabilitation Act of 1973 or for improved design for patients with cognitive disabilities. Refer to the CMS website on section 508 of the Rehabilitation Act (https://www.cms.gov/Research-Statistics-Data-and- Systems/CMS-Information- Technology/Section508/index.html?redirect=/InfoTech GenInfo/07_Section508.asp) that requires institutions receiving federal funds to solicit, procure, maintain, and use all electronic and information technology (EIT) so that equal or alternate/comparable access is given to members of the public with and without disabilities. For example, this includes designing a patient portal or website that is compliant with section 508 of the Rehabilitation Act of 1973.	Medium	IA_BE_5
Beneficiary Engagement	Collection and Follow-Up on Patient Experience and Satisfaction Data on Beneficiary Engagement Collection and follow-up on patient experience and satisfaction data on beneficiary engagement, including development of improvement plan.	High	IA_BE_6
Beneficiary Engagement	Participation in a QCDR, that promotes use of patient engagement tools.	Medium	IA_BE_7
Beneficiary Engagement	Participation in a QCDR, that promotes collaborative learning network opportunities that are interactive.	Medium	IA_BE_8
Beneficiary Engagement	Use of QCDR patient experience data to inform and advance improvements in beneficiary engagement.	Medium	IA_BE_9
Beneficiary Engagement	Participation in a QCDR, that promotes implementation of patient self-action plans.	Medium	IA_BE_10
Beneficiary Engagement	Participation in a QCDR, that promotes use of processes and tools that engage patients for adherence to treatment plan.	Medium	IA_BE_11
Beneficiary Engagement	Use evidence-based decision aids to support shared decision making.	Medium	IA_BE_12
Beneficiary Engagement	Regularly assess the patient experience of care through surveys, advisory councils, and/or other mechanisms.	Medium	IA_BE_13

(continued on next page)

TABLE 3-26. List of Improvement Activities (continued)

Subcategory	Activity Title + Description	Weight	Activity ID
Beneficiary Engagement	**Engage Patients and Families to Guide Improvement in the System of Care** Engage patients and families to guide improvement in the system of care by leveraging digital tools for ongoing guidance and assessments outside the encounter, including the collection and use of patient data for return-to-work and patient quality of life improvement. Platforms and devices that collect patient-generated health data (PGHD) must do so with an active feedback loop, either providing PGHD in real or near-real time to the care team, or generating clinically endorsed real or near-real time automated feedback to the patient, including patient-reported outcomes (PROs). Examples include patient engagement and outcomes tracking platforms, cellular or web-enabled bi- directional systems, and other devices that transmit clinically valid objective and subjective data back to care teams. Because many consumer-grade devices capture PGHD (for example, wellness devices), platforms or devices eligible for this improvement activity must be, at a minimum, endorsed and offered clinically by care teams to patients to automatically send ongoing guidance (one way). Platforms and devices that additionally collect PGHD must do so with an active feedback loop, either providing PGHD in real or near-real time to the care team, or generating clinically endorsed real or near-real time automated feedback to the patient (e.g. automated patient-facing instructions based on glucometer readings). Therefore, unlike passive platforms or devices that may collect but do not transmit PGHD in real or near-real time to clinical care teams, active devices and platforms can inform the patient or the clinical care team in a timely manner of important parameters regarding a patient's status, adherence, comprehension, and indicators of clinical concern.	High	IA_BE_14
Beneficiary Engagement	**Engage Patients, Family, and Caregivers in Developing a Plan of Care** Engage patients, family and caregivers in developing a plan of care and prioritizing their goals for action, documented in the certified EHR technology.	Medium	IA_BE_15
Beneficiary Engagement	**Evidenced-Based Techniques to Promote Self-Management into Usual Care** Incorporate evidence-based techniques to promote self-management into usual care, leveraging techniques such as goal setting with structured follow-up, teach back, action planning, or motivational interviewing.	Medium	IA_BE_16
Beneficiary Engagement	**Use of Tools to Assist Patient Self-Management** Use tools to assist patients in assessing their need for support for self-management (e.g., the Patient Activation Measure or How's My Health).	Medium	IA_BE_17
Beneficiary Engagement	Provide peer-led support for self-management.	Medium	IA_BE_18
Beneficiary Engagement	Use group visits for common chronic conditions (e.g., diabetes).	Medium	IA_BE_19
Beneficiary Engagement	**Implementation of Condition-Specific Chronic Disease Self-Management Support Programs** Provide condition-specific chronic disease self-management support programs or coaching, or link patients to those programs in the community.	Medium	IA_BE_20
Beneficiary Engagement	**Improved Practices that Disseminate Appropriate Self-Management Materials** Provide self-management materials at an appropriate literacy level and in an appropriate language.	Medium	IA_BE_21

(continued on next page)

TABLE 3-26. List of Improvement Activities (continued)

Subcategory	Activity Title + Description	Weight	Activity ID
Beneficiary Engagement	Improved Practices that Engage Patients Pre-Visit Implement workflow changes that engage patients prior to the visit, such as a pre-visit development of a shared visit agenda with the patient, or targeted pre-visit laboratory testing that will be resulted and available to the MIPS-eligible clinician to review and discuss during the patient's appointment.	Medium	IA_BE_22
Beneficiary Engagement	Integration of Patient Coaching Practices between Visits Provide coaching between visits with follow-up on care plan and goals.	Medium	IA_BE_23
Patient Safety and Practice Assessment	Participation in an AHRQ-listed patient safety organization.	Medium	IA_PSPA_1
Patient Safety and Practice Assessment	Participation in MOC Part IV Participation in Maintenance of Certification (MOC) Part IV, such as the American Board of Internal Medicine (ABIM) Approved Quality Improvement (AQI) Program, National Cardiovascular Data Registry (NCDR) Clinical Quality Coach, Quality Practice Initiative Certification Program, American Board of Medical Specialties Practice Performance Improvement Module, or ASA Simulation Education Network, for improving professional practice including participation in a local, regional or national outcomes registry or quality assessment program. Perform monthly activities across practice to regularly assess performance in practice by reviewing outcomes addressing identified areas for improvement and evaluating the results.	Medium	IA_PSPA_2
Patient Safety and Practice Assessment	Participate in IHI Training/Forum Event (e.g., National Academy of Medicine, AHRQ Team STEPPS® or Similar Activity) For MIPS-eligible clinicians not participating in Maintenance of Certification (MOC) Part IV, new engagement for MOC Part IV, such as the Institute for Healthcare Improvement (IHI) Training/Forum Event, National Academy of Medicine, Agency for Healthcare Research and Quality (AHRQ) Team STEPPS®, or the American Board of Family Medicine (ABFM) Performance in Practice Modules.	Medium	IA_PSPA_3
Patient Safety and Practice Assessment	Administration of the AHRQ Survey of Patient Safety Culture Administration of the AHRQ Survey of Patient Safety Culture and submission of data to the comparative database (refer to AHRQ Survey of Patient Safety Culture website: http://www.ahrq.gov/professionals/quality-patient- safety/patientsafetyculture/index.html). **Note:** This activity may be selected once every four years to avoid duplicative information since some of the modules may change on a year by year basis, but over four years there would be a reasonable expectation for the set of modules to have undergone substantive change for the improvement activities performance category score.	Medium	IA_PSPA_4
Patient Safety and Practice Assessment	Annual Registration in the Prescription Drug Monitoring Program Annual registration by eligible clinician or group in the prescription drug-monitoring program of the state where she practices. Activities that simply involve registration are not sufficient. MIPS-eligible clinicians and groups must participate for a minimum of six months.	Medium	IA_PSPA_5

(continued on next page)

TABLE 3-26. List of Improvement Activities (continued)

Subcategory	Activity Title + Description	Weight	Activity ID
Patient Safety and Practice Assessment	Consultation of the Prescription Drug Monitoring program Clinicians would attest to reviewing the patient's history of controlled substance prescription using state prescription drug monitoring program (PDMP) data prior to the issuance of a Controlled Substance Schedule II (CSII) opioid prescription lasting longer than three days. For the transition year, clinicians would attest to a 60 percent review of applicable patient's history. For the Quality Payment Program Year 2 and future years, clinicians would attest to a 75 percent review of applicable patient's history performance.	High	IA_PSPA_6
Patient Safety and Practice Assessment	Use of QCDR Data for Ongoing Practice Assessment and Improvements Use of QCDR data, for ongoing practice assessment, and improvements in patient safety.	Medium	IA_PSPA_7
Patient Safety and Practice Assessment	Use of Patient Safety Tools Use of tools that assist specialty practices in tracking specific measures that are meaningful to their practice—such as use of a surgical risk calculator, evidence based protocols such as Enhanced Recovery After Surgery (ERAS) protocols, the CDC Guide for Infection Prevention for Outpatient Settings, (https://www.cdc.gov/hai/settings/outpatient/outpatient-care-guidelines.html), predictive algorithms, or other such tools.	Medium	IA_PSPA_8
Patient Safety and Practice Assessment	Completion of the American Medical Association's STEPS Forward program.	Medium	IA_PSPA_9
Patient Safety and Practice Assessment	Completion of Training and Receipt of Approved Waiver for Provision Opioid Medication-Assisted Treatments Completion of training and obtaining an approved waiver for provision of medication-assisted treatment of opioid use disorders using buprenorphine.	Medium	IA_PSPA_10
Patient Safety and Practice Assessment	Participation in CAHPS or Other Supplemental Questionnaire Participation in the Consumer Assessment of Healthcare Providers and Systems Survey or other supplemental questionnaire items (e.g., Cultural Competence or Health Information Technology supplemental item sets).	High	IA_PSPA_11
Patient Safety and Practice Assessment	Participation in Private Payer CPIA Participation in designated private payer clinical practice improvement activities.	Medium	IA_PSPA_12
Patient Safety and Practice Assessment	Participation in Joint Commission Ongoing Professional Practice Evaluation initiative.	Medium	IA_PSPA_13
Patient Safety and Practice Assessment	Participation in Bridges to Excellence or Other Similar Program Participation in quality improvement programs such as Bridges to Excellence or American Board of Medical Specialties (ABMS) Multi-Specialty Portfolio Program.	Medium	IA_PSPA_14
Patient Safety and Practice Assessment	Implementation of Antibiotic Stewardship Program Implementation of an antibiotic stewardship program that measures the appropriate use of antibiotics for several different conditions (eg. URI Rx in children, diagnosis of pharyngitis, Bronchitis Rx in adults) according to clinical guidelines for diagnostics and therapeutics.	Medium	IA_PSPA_15

(continued on next page)

TABLE 3-26. List of Improvement Activities (continued)

Subcategory	Activity Title + Description	Weight	Activity ID
Patient Safety and Practice Assessment	Use decision support and standardized treatment protocols to manage workflow in the team to meet patient needs.	Medium	IA_PSPA_16
Patient Safety and Practice Assessment	Implementation of Analytic Capabilities to Manage Total Cost of Care for Practice Population Build the analytic capability required to manage total cost of care for the practice population that could include one or more of the following: • Train appropriate staff on interpretation of cost and utilization information; and/or • Use available data regularly to analyze opportunities to reduce cost through improved care.	Medium	IA_PSPA_17
Patient Safety and Practice Assessment	Measurement and Improvement at the Practice and Panel Levels Measure and improve quality at the practice and panel levels, such as implementing the American Board of Orthopaedic Surgery (ABOS) Physician Scorecards, that could include one or more of the following: • Regularly review measures of quality, utilization, patient satisfaction, and other measures that may be useful at the practice level and at the level of the care team or MIPS-eligible clinician or group (panel); and/or • Use relevant data sources to create benchmarks and goals for performance at the practice level and panel level.	Medium	IA_PSPA_18
Patient Safety and Practice Assessment	Implementation of Formal Quality Improvement Methods, Practice Changes, or Other Practice Improvement Processes Adopt a formal model for quality improvement and create a culture in which all staff actively participate in improvement activities that could include one or more of the following such as: • Multi-Source Feedback; • Train all staff in quality improvement methods; • Integrate practice change/quality improvement into staff duties; • Engage all staff in identifying and testing practices changes; • Designate regular team meetings to review data and plan improvement cycles; • Promote transparency and accelerate improvement by sharing practice level and panel level quality of care, patient experience and utilization data with staff; and/or • Promote transparency and engage patients and families by sharing practice-level quality of care, patient experience, and utilization data with patients and families, including activities in which clinicians act upon patient experience data.	Medium	IA_PSPA_19
Patient Safety and Practice Assessment	Leadership Engagement in Regular Guidance and Demonstrated Commitment for Implementing Practice Improvement Changes Ensure full engagement of clinical and administrative leadership in practice improvement that could include one or more of the following: • Make responsibility for guidance of practice change a component of clinical and administrative leadership roles; • Allocate time for clinical and administrative leadership for practice improvement efforts, including participation in regular team meetings; and/or • Incorporate population health, quality, and patient experience metrics in regular reviews of practice performance.	Medium	IA_PSPA_20

(continued on next page)

TABLE 3-26. List of Improvement Activities (continued)

Subcategory	Activity Title + Description	Weight	Activity ID
Patient Safety and Practice Assessment	Implementation of Fall Screening and Assessment Programs Implementation of fall screening and assessment programs to identify patients at risk for falls and address modifiable risk factors (e.g., clinical decision support/prompts in the electronic health record that help manage the use of medications that increase fall risk, such as benzodiazepines).	Medium	IA_PSPA_21
Patient Safety and Practice Assessment	CDC training on CDC's Guideline for Prescribing Opioids for Chronic Pain Completion of all the modules of the Centers for Disease Control and Prevention (CDC) course "Applying CDC's Guideline for Prescribing Opioids" that reviews the 2016 "Guideline for Prescribing Opioids for Chronic Pain." **Note:** This activity may be selected once every four years to avoid duplicative information given that some of the modules may change on a year by year basis, since over four years there would be a reasonable expectation for the set of modules to have undergone substantive change for the improvement activities performance category score.	High	IA_PSPA_22
Patient Safety and Practice Assessment	Initiate CDC Training on Antibiotic Stewardship Complete more than 50 percent of the modules of the Centers for Disease Control and Prevention antibiotic stewardship course. **Note:** This activity may be selected once every four years to avoid duplicative information given that some of the modules may change on a year by year basis, since over four years there would be a reasonable expectation for the set of modules to have undergone substantive change for the improvement activities performance category score.	Medium	IA_PSPA_24
Patient Safety and Practice Assessment	Cost Display for Laboratory and Radiographic Orders Implementation of a cost display for laboratory and radiographic orders, such as costs that can be obtained through the Medicare clinical laboratory fee schedule.	Medium	IA_PSPA_25
Patient Safety and Practice Assessment	Communication of Unscheduled Visit for Adverse Drug Event and Nature of Event A MIPS-eligible clinician provides unscheduled care (such as an emergency room, urgent care, or other unplanned encounter) and attests that for greater than 75 percent of case visits that result from a clinically significant adverse drug event, the MIPS-eligible clinician provides information, including through the use of health IT to the patient's primary care clinician regarding both the unscheduled visit and the nature of the adverse drug event within 48 hours. A clinically significant adverse event is defined as a medication-related harm or injury such as side effects, supratherapeutic effects, allergic reactions, laboratory abnormalities, or medication errors requiring urgent/emergent evaluation, treatment, or hospitalization.	Medium	IA_PSPA_26
Patient Safety and Practice Assessment	Invasive Procedure or Surgery Anticoagulation Medication Management For an anticoagulated patient undergoing a planned invasive procedure for which interruption in anticoagulation is anticipated, including patients taking vitamin K antagonists (warfarin), target specific oral anticoagulants (such as apixaban, dabigatran, and rivaroxaban), and heparins/low molecular weight heparins, documentation, including through the use of electronic tools, ensuring that the plan for anticoagulation management in the periprocedural period was discussed with the patient and with the clinician responsible for managing the patient's anticoagulation. Elements of the plan should include the following: discontinuation, resumption, and, if applicable, bridging, laboratory monitoring, and management of concomitant antithrombotic medications (such as antiplatelets and nonsteroidalanti-inflammatory drugs (NSAIDs)). An invasive or surgical procedure is defined as a procedure in which skin or mucous membranes and connective tissue are incised, or an instrument is introduced through a natural body orifice.	Medium	IA_PSPA_27

(continued on next page)

TABLE 3-26. List of Improvement Activities (continued)

Subcategory	Activity Title + Description	Weight	Activity ID
Patient Safety and Practice Assessment	Completion of an Accredited Safety or Quality Improvement Program Complete an accredited performance improvement continuing medical education program that addresses performance or quality improvement according to the following criteria: • The activity must address a quality or safety gap that is supported by a needs assessment or problem analysis, or must support the completion of such a needs assessment as part of the activity; • The activity must have specific, measurable aim(s) for improvement; • The activity must include interventions intended to result in improvement; • The activity must include data collection and analysis of performance data to assess the impact of the interventions; and • The accredited program must define meaningful clinician participation in its activity, describe the mechanism for identifying clinicians who meet the requirements, and provide participant completion information.	Medium	IA_PSPA_28
Patient Safety and Practice Assessment	Consulting AUC Using Clinical Decision Support When Ordering Advanced Clinicians attest that they are consulting specified applicable AUC through a qualified clinical decision support mechanism for all applicable imaging services furnished in an applicable setting, paid for under an applicable payment system, and ordered on or after January 1, 2018. This activity is for clinicians that are early adopters of the Medicare AUC program (2018 performance year) and for clinicians that begin the Medicare AUC program in future years as specified in our regulation at §414.94. The AUC program is required under section 218 of the Protecting Access to Medicare Act of 2014. Qualified mechanisms will be able to provide a report to the ordering clinician that can be used to assess patterns of image-ordering and improve upon those patterns to ensure that patients are receiving the most appropriate imaging for their individual condition.	High	IA_PSPA_29
Patient Safety and Practice Assessment	PCI Bleeding Campaign Participate in the PCI Bleeding Campaign, which is a national quality improvement program that provides infrastructure for a learning network and offers evidence-based resources and tools to reduce avoidable bleeding associated with patients who receive a percutaneous coronary intervention (PCI). The program uses a patient-centered and team-based approach, leveraging evidence-based best practices to improve care for PCI patients by implementing quality improvement strategies: • Radial-artery access, • Bivalirudin, and • Use of vascular closure devices.	High	IA_PSPA_30
Achieving Health Equity	Engagement of New Medicaid Patients and Follow-Up Seeing new and follow-up Medicaid patients in a timely manner, including individuals dually eligible for Medicaid and Medicare. A timely manner is defined as within 10 business days for this activity.	High	IA_AHE_1
Achieving Health Equity	Leveraging a QCDR to Standardize Processes for Screening Participate in a QCDR, demonstrating performance of activities for use of standardized processes for screening for social determinants of health such as food security, employment, and housing. Use of supporting tools that can be incorporated into the certified EHR technology is also suggested.	Medium	IA_AHE_2

(continued on next page)

TABLE 3-26. List of Improvement Activities (continued)

Subcategory	Activity Title + Description	Weight	Activity ID
Achieving Health Equity	Leveraging a QCDR to Promote Use of Patient-Reported Outcome Tools Participation in a QCDR, demonstrating performance of activities for employing patient-reported outcome (PRO) tools and corresponding collection of PRO data such as the use of PQH-2 or PHQ-9, PROMIS instruments, patient reported Wound-Quality of Life (QoL), patient-reported Wound Outcome, and patient-reported Nutritional Screening.	High	IA_AHE_3
Achieving Health Equity	Leveraging a QCDR for Use of Standard Questionnaires Participate in a QCDR, demonstrating performance of activities for use of standard questionnaires for assessing improvements in health disparities related to functional health status (e.g., use of Seattle Angina Questionnaire, MD Anderson Symptom Inventory, and/or SF-12/VR-12 functional health status assessment).	Medium	IA_AHE_4
Achieving Health Equity	MIPS-Eligible Clinician Leadership in Clinical Trials or CBPR Initiate MIPS-eligible clinician leadership in clinical trials, research alliances, or community-based participatory research (CBPR) that identify tools, research, or processes that can focuses on minimizing disparities in healthcare access, care quality, affordability, or outcomes.	Medium	IA_AHE_5
Achieving Health Equity	Provide Education Opportunities for New Clinicians MIPS-eligible clinicians acting as a preceptor for clinicians-in-training (such as medical residents/fellows, medical students, physician assistants, nurse practitioners, or clinical nurse specialists) should accept such clinicians for clinical rotations in community practices in small, underserved, or rural areas.	High	IA_AHE_6
Emergency Response and Preparedness	Participation on Disaster Medical Assistance Team, Registered for 6 Months Participate in Disaster Medical Assistance Teams or Community Emergency Responder Teams. Activities that simply involve registration are not sufficient. MIPS-eligible clinicians and MIPS-eligible clinician groups must be registered for a minimum of six months as a volunteer for disaster or emergency response.	Medium	IA_ERP_1
Emergency Response and Preparedness	Participation in a 60-Day or Greater Effort to Support Domestic or International Humanitarian Needs Participate in domestic or international humanitarian volunteer work. Activities that simply involve registration are not sufficient. MIPS-eligible clinicians and groups attest to domestic or international humanitarian volunteer work for a period of a continuous 60 days or longer.	High	IA_ERP_2
Behavioral and Mental Health	Diabetes Screening Conduct diabetes screening for people with schizophrenia or bipolar disease who are using antipsychotic medication.	Medium	IA_BMH_1
Behavioral and Mental Health	Tobacco Use Regular engagement of MIPS-eligible clinicians or groups in integrated prevention and treatment interventions, including tobacco use screening and cessation interventions (refer to NQF #0028) for patients with co-occurring conditions of behavioral or mental health and at-risk factors for tobacco dependence.	Medium	IA_BMH_2
Behavioral and Mental Health	Unhealthy Alcohol Use Regular engagement of MIPS-eligible clinicians or groups in integrated prevention and treatment interventions, including screening and brief counseling (refer to NQF #2152) for patients with co-occurring conditions of behavioral or mental health conditions.	Medium	IA_BMH_3

(continued on next page)

TABLE 3-26. List of Improvement Activities (continued)

Subcategory	Activity Title + Description	Weight	Activity ID
Behavioral and Mental Health	**Depression Screening** Depression Screening and Follow-Up Plan: Regular engagement of MIPS-eligible clinicians or groups in integrated prevention and treatment interventions, including depression screening, and follow-up plan (refer to NQF #0418) for patients with co-occurring conditions of behavioral or mental health conditions.	Medium	IA_BMH_4
Behavioral and Mental Health	**MDD Prevention and Treatment Interventions** Major Depressive Disorder: Regular engagement of MIPS-eligible clinicians or groups in integrated prevention and treatment interventions, including suicide risk assessment (refer to NQF #0104) for mental health patients with co-occurring conditions of behavioral or mental health conditions.	Medium	IA_BMH_5
Behavioral and Mental Health	**Implementation of Co-Location PCP and MH Services** Promote integration facilitation and the colocation of mental health and substance use disorder services in primary and/or non-primary clinical care settings.	High	IA_BMH_6
Behavioral and Mental Health	**Implementation of Integrated Patient Centered Behavioral Health (PCBH) Model** Offer integrated behavioral health services to support patients with behavioral health needs who also have conditions such as dementia or other poorly controlled chronic illnesses. The services could include one or more of the following: • Use evidence-based treatment protocols and treatment to goal where appropriate; • Use evidence-based screening and case finding strategies to identify individuals at risk and in need of services; • Ensure regular communication and coordinated workflows between MIPS-eligible clinicians in primary care and behavioral health; • Conduct regular case reviews for at-risk or unstable patients and those who are not responding to treatment; • Use a registry or health information technology functionality to support active care management and outreach to patients in treatment; • Integrate behavioral health and medical care plans and facilitate integration through co-location of services when feasible; and/or • Participate in the National Partnership to Improve Dementia Care Initiative, which promotes a multidimensional approach that includes public reporting, state-based coalitions, research, training, and revised survey or guidance.	High	IA_BMH_7
Behavioral and Mental Health	**Electronic Health Record Enhancements for BH Data Capture** Contribute enhancements to an electronic health record to capture additional data on behavioral health (BH) populations and use that data for additional decision making purposes (e.g., capture of additional BH data results in additional depression screening for at-risk patient not previously identified).	Medium	IA_BMH_8
Behavioral and Mental Health	**Unhealthy Alcohol Use for Patients with Co-Occurring Conditions of Mental Health and Substance Abuse and Ambulatory Care Patients** Individual MIPS-eligible clinicians or groups must regularly engage in integrated prevention and treatment interventions, including screening and brief counseling (for example: NQF #2152) for patients with co-occurring conditions of mental health and substance abuse. MIPS-eligible clinicians would attest that 60 percent for the CY 2018 Quality Payment Program performance period, and 75 percent beginning in the 2019 performance period, of their ambulatory care patients are screened for unhealthy alcohol use.	High	IA_BMH_9

Score

The improvement activities performance category will account for 15 percent of the final score, dependent on group size (Figure 3-23).

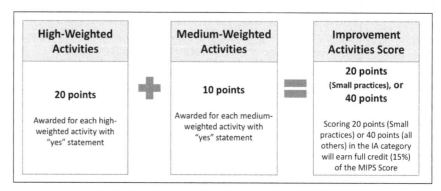

FIGURE 3-23. Scoring the Improvement Activity Category

Groups with 16 or More Clinicians

To receive the maximum points available for this category, groups with 16 or more clinicians can earn up to 40 points by completing up to four improvement activities for a minimum of 90 days.

Each activity is weighted as "medium" or "high." To get the maximum score of 40 points for the Improvement Activity score, you may select any of these combinations:

- Two high-weighted activities
- One high-weighted activity and two medium-weighted activities
- Up to four medium-weighted activities

Each medium-weighted activity is worth 10 points of the total Improvement Activity performance category score, and each high-weighted activity is worth 20 points of the total category score.

If you are not participating in an APM, a certified patient-centered medical home or comparable specialty practice, and you do not select any activities, you will receive 0 points in this performance category.

Groups with 15 or Fewer Clinicians, Non-Patient Facing Clinicians and/or Clinicians Located in a Rural Area or HPSA

To receive the maximum points available for this category, groups of fewer than 15 clinicians can earn up to 20 points by completing up to two improvement activities for a minimum of 90 days.

Again, each activity is weighted either "medium" or "high." To achieve the maximum 20 points for the Improvement Activity score, you may select either of these combinations:

- One high-weighted activity
- Two medium-weighted activities

These clinicians may select two medium-weighted activities or one high-weighted activity to receive a total of 20 points of the total category score.

Participants in certified patient-centered medical homes, comparable specialty practices, or an APM designated as a Medical Home Model, will automatically earn full credit.

Participants in certain APMs under the APM scoring standard, such as Shared Savings Program Track 1 or OCM, will automatically be scored based on the requirements of participating in the APM. For all current APMs under the APM scoring standard, this assigned score will constitute full credit. For all future APMs under the APM scoring standard, the assigned score will be at least half credit.

Participants in any other APM will automatically earn half credit and may report additional activities to increase the score.

Keys to Success

- Select four or more possible activities. You may want to select more than the minimum for your practice size because you may find that some activities are easier to implement than others.
- Look for things you may be doing already that would earn points.
- An EHR is not required for many of the activities. However, some are best suited to an EHR or your EHR may support the activity. Check with your vendor.
- Document the process for each activity, making sure to include how and when the activity took place, and also making sure to demonstrate that each activity is in place for at least 90 days.
- Implement/adjust your process for each activity as necessary. Hold at least one meeting with your staff to ensure the activity is in place and working properly, making sure to document that the meeting took place.
- For any improvement activity, you select, you must be prepared to prove that you have done the activity if audited by CMS.

Resources

- https://qpp.cms.gov/mips/improvement-activities
- https://www.cms.gov/Medicare/Quality-Payment-Program/Resource-Library/2018-Resources.html

The QPP resource library has a document titled "MIPS Data Validation Criteria" that lists the type of documentation you would be expected to supply to CMS in case of an audit.

Lessons Learned from the Field

Lesson 1: Double dip if you can!

Oftentimes, an improvement activity can align something you're already doing with something you want to do in the future. In some cases, for example, activities that involve a QCDR can earn points in multiple categories.

If you choose an activity that represents something you're already doing, then you may just need to officially document the processes that you already have in place.

CALCULATING THE COMPOSITE PERFORMANCE SCORE

As you know by now, MIPS is a comparative and competitive program in which the Composite Performance Score will be the primary determinant of payment adjustments.

Whether reporting as an individual, a group, a virtual group, or a MIPS APM, CMS goes through these six steps to determine the MIPS payment adjustment:

1. Data submission
2. Category scoring
3. Composite Performance Score (CPS) calculation [Range 0-100]
4. CPS comparison with CPS performance threshold
5. Payment adjustment determination and scaling
6. Payment adjustment application

Once data has been submitted to CMS, the calculation of the payment adjustment under MIPS starts with a clinician receiving a performance category score and then multiplying that score by the weight assigned to the performance category.

After scoring the four performance categories, CMS takes into account the size of the practice and the complexity of the clinician's patients (Figure 3-24).

Small Practice Bonus

CMS will add five bonus points to the final score for MIPS-eligible clinicians, groups, APM Entities, and virtual groups that meet the definition of a small practice and submit data on at least one performance category in the 2018 performance period.

Remember, the definition of a small practice for the 2018 performance year is a practice with 15 or fewer eligible clinicians, using claims data from

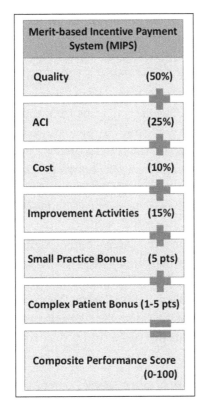

FIGURE 3-24. Calculating the MIPS Complete Performance Score

Sept 1, 2016 to Aug 31, 2017, plus a 30-day claims run out to determine which practices will be deemed "small."

Complex Patient Bonus

Clinicians who care for sicker patients, understandably, don't want their scores to be hurt due to conditions that are beyond their control. CMS recognized this through provider feedback and to address this, they will add up to five bonus points to the final score for MIPS-eligible clinicians, groups, APM Entities, and virtual groups that submit data for at least one MIPS performance category during the 2018 performance period.

CMS identified two potential indicators for complexity: medical complexity as measured through Hierarchical Condition Category (HCC) risk scores, and social risk as measured through the proportion of patients with dual eligible status. Both of these indicators have been used in Medicare programs to account for risk and both data elements are already publicly available.

"Dual eligible" is the general term that describes individuals who are enrolled in both Medicare and Medicaid. The term includes individuals who are enrolled in Medicare Part A and/or Part B and receive full Medicaid benefits and/or assistance with Medicare premiums or cost sharing through a "Medicare Savings Program" category.

The dual eligibility ratio will be calculated based on the proportion of unique patients who have dual eligible status seen by the MIPS-eligible clinician among all unique patients seen during the second 12-month segment of the eligibility period. This period spans from the last four months of a calendar year that is one year prior (i.e. September 1—August 31). This is the same time period used for the HCC score.

To calculate the complex patient bonus for *individual clinicians* and *groups*, CMS will add the average HCC risk score to the dual eligible ratio, based on full benefit and partial benefit dual eligible beneficiaries, multiplied by five.

To calculate the complex patient bonus for *APM Entities* and *virtual groups*, CMS will add the beneficiary weighted average HCC risk score for all MIPS-eligible clinicians to the average dual eligible ratio for all MIPS-eligible clinicians, multiplied by five. If it's technically feasible, CMS will do the same for TINs for models and virtual groups which rely on complete TIN participation, within the APM Entity or virtual group, respectively (Table 3-27).

TABLE 3-27. Average HCC Risk Score by Practice Size

Practice Size	Average HCC Risk Score	Dual Eligible Ratio
1-15 clinicians	1.61	24.90%
16-24 clinicians	1.70	26.20%
25-99 clinicians	1.72	27.50%
100+ clinicians	1.82	26.90%
Average	1.75	26.60%

A few things to remember:

A clinician's or group's payment adjustment will not be a set amount, but is determined by the score. It is a percentage of a provider's Medicare Part-B billings. So the reward and penalty will not be identical for everyone. Higher scores will earn a higher positive adjustment percentage.

Earning a particular score will not guarantee you a certain bonus. Expect there to be a fair distribution of the available monies among all in that score segment.

Prepare yourself. The thresholds will move every year. The 2017 performance year had low thresholds and category score requirements only because it was the transition year. Requirements have already gotten tougher and thresholds are higher; we expect this trend to continue.

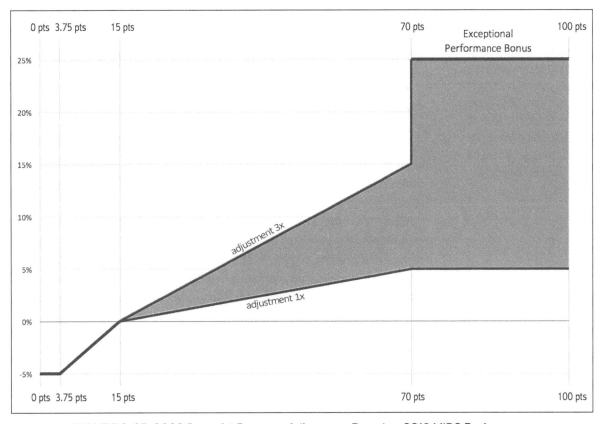

FIGURE 3-25. 2020 Potential Payment Adjustment Based on 2018 MIPS Performance

Although MIPS is a budget-neutral program, there is an additional $500 million annual budget allocated from year 2019 through 2024 to incentivize exceptional performers. So MIPS participants can earn two types of payment adjustments:

1. **Budget Neutral Payment Adjustment**—All the money collected as penalties (negative payment adjustments) will be distributed as positive payment adjustments (-5% to +5% of your 2020 Medicare Part-B Billings)

2. **Exceptional Performance Payment Adjustment**—A $500 Million annual budget will be utilized for additional positive payment adjustment, topping the budget-neutral payment adjustment that exceptional performers can earn (up to 10% of your Medicare Part-B Billings).

Based on your MIPS Score (CPS), you will earn either a positive payment adjustment or a negative payment adjustment. Here is a simplified representation of the payment adjustment distribution based on 2018 Performance Year scores for Payment Year 2020 (Figure 3-25).

Although you can't control what percentage you would earn for positive payment adjustments, you can definitely take charge of your MIPS Score and be proactive about it. Understand where you stand today and what you need to be your best.

CPS 0—3.75: Maximum negative payment adjustment (-5%) will apply.

CPS 3.76—14.99: Negative payment adjustment gradually decreases on a linear sliding scale from -5% to 0% will apply.

CPS 15: Payment adjustment of zero percent.

CPS 15.01—69.99: Providers will receive the budget-neutral component of positive payment adjustment, which is scaled from zero to five percent. A scaling factor (up to a max of three) will be used to equitably distribute every single cent of the penalties collected. It means that there is a potential to earn a maximum of 15 percent positive adjustment, provided there is enough money collected as penalties.

CPS 70—100: The providers whose scores lie in this range, will earn the same positive payment described above, plus an additional exceptional performance positive payment adjustment. This bonus will be distributed from the $500 million annual budget up to a max of +10% even if there is money left over. Another scaling factor will be utilized to ensure a fair distribution of the monies, for example more money for a higher score while staying within the annual budget of $500 million.

Although you can't control what percentage you would earn for positive payment adjustments, you can definitely take charge of your MIPS Score and be proactive about it. Understand where you stand today and what you need to be your best.

CHAPTER 4

Reporting Your Data

Data submission mechanisms for MIPS-eligible clinicians reporting individually include the following:

MIPS ECs reporting as individuals will have the option to report the quality, advancing care information, and improvement activity categories by QCDR, registry, or by EHR—depending on what is technically feasible and according to their preference.

They also have the option to report quality measures via claims. However, note that not all quality measures are available for claims reporting.

The cost category does not require submission by an eligible clinician, since it is calculated by CMS when providers submit their claims data (Table 4-1).

TABLE 4-1. Submission Mechanisms Available for Each Performance Category for Clinicians Reporting as an Individual

Performance Category/Submission Combinations Accepted	Individual Reporting Data Submission Mechanisms
Quality	Claims QCDR Registry EHR
Advancing Care Information	Attestation QCDR Registry EHR
Cost	Administrative Claims (no submission required)
Improvement Activities	Attestation QCDR Registry EHR

Data Submission Mechanisms for MIPS-Eligible Clinicians Reporting as Groups (TIN)

MIPS ECs who report as a group will have the option to report quality, advancing care information, and improvement activities by QCDR, registry, EHR, or

CMS Web Interface (groups of 25 or more)—depending on what is technically feasible and according to their preference.

CMS will calculate the cost category and the all-cause readmission measure for them (Table 4-2).

TABLE 4-2. Submission Mechanisms Available for Each Performance Category for Clinicians Reporting as a Group

Performance Category/Submission Combinations Accepted	Individual Reporting Data Submission Mechanisms
Quality	QCDR Registry EHR CMS Web Interface (groups of 25+ ECs) CMS-approved survey vendor for CAHPS for MIPS (must be reported in conjunction with another data submission mechanism) Administrative claims (for all-cause hospital readmission measure; no submission required)
Advancing Care Information	Attestation QCDR Registry EHR CMS Web Interface (groups of 25+ ECs)
Cost	Administrative Claims
Improvement Activities	Attestation QCDR Registry EHR CMS Web Interface (groups of 25+ ECs)

ENTERPRISE IDENTITY DATA MANAGEMENT ACCOUNT

Clinicians, groups, MIPS APMs, and certain Advanced APM participants, will need an Enterprise Identity Data Management (EIDM) account with a role under the "Physician Quality and Value Programs" section if they intend to do any of the following (see Figure 4-1. Login Page to QPP Attestation System and Table 4-3. EIDM Reporting Options):

- Submit data directly to *qpp.cms.gov*.
- Have an EHR/Health IT vendor submit their data to *qpp.cms.gov* on their behalf.
- View or be able to view the data submitted on their behalf by a third party.

QCDRs, registries, and EHR/Health IT vendors must also have an EIDM account with a role tied to the "Physician Quality and Value Pro-

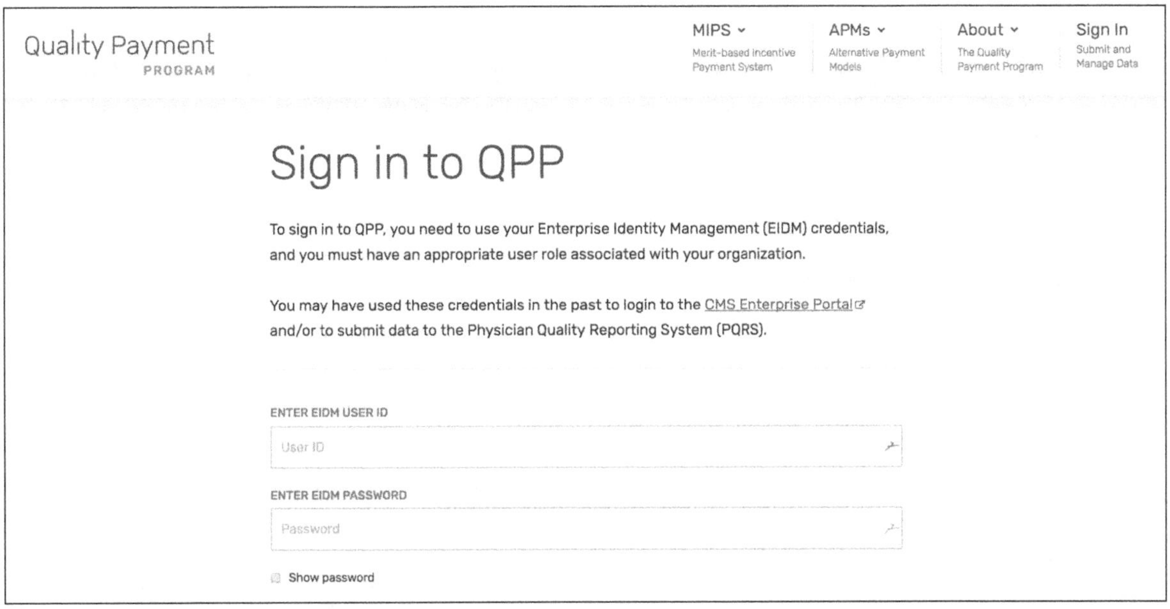

FIGURE 4-1. Login Page to QPP Attestation System

grams" to be able to submit data directly to *qpp.cms.gov* on behalf of their clients.

All EIDM account holders must be in the United States of America.

The information provided below was accurate for the 2017 performance year. Details will likely be updated by CMS for the 2018 performance year, but in the spirit of sharing the available information to let you know what to expect, well, here you go (Table 4-4).

To submit data directly to QPP, users will need to request the same roles that were needed to submit data to the Physician Quality Reporting System (PQRS). Please note: Even though the EIDM naming convention still refers to "PQRS," these are the roles needed for QPP submission.

Your Attestation Prep To-Do List:

1. Determine whether your organization is already registered in EIDM.
2. Identify your organization's Security Official. If your group does not already have one, designate one!
3. Gather the required information for each role.
   - Users requesting the **Security Official** role must provide all of the following:
     — Group's Medicare billing TIN
     — Legal Business Name
     — Rendering NPIs for two different eligible clinicians who bill under the TIN and their corresponding individual Provider Transaction

TABLE 4-3. EIDM Reporting Options

Reporting Option	Purpose

Groups, including:
• MIPS APM participants
• Non-QP Advanced APM participants
(2+ clinicians billing under the TIN)
	1. Group or clinician representatives that will be **submitting MIPS data directly** to qpp.cms.gov including data for any, or all, of the following MIPS performance categories (individual or group reporting):
	  • Quality (via file upload or CMS Web Interface)
	  • Advancing Care Information (via file upload, attestation, or CMS Web Interface)
	  • Improvement Activities (via file upload, attestation, or CMS Web Interface)
	IMPORTANT! Groups participating in a Shared Savings Program (SSP) ACO must obtain EIDM accounts and roles to submit and meet the Advancing Care Information requirements under MIPS for purposes of the MIPS APM Scoring Standard and the Shared Savings Program ACO-11 quality measure.
	2. Groups, reporting as individuals or a group, that **have secured an EHR/Health IT Vendor to submit data on their behalf** (those that are not a CMS-approved Qualified Clinical Data Registry or Qualified Registry)
	3. Group representatives that want to **view data submitted on their behalf** (reporting as individuals or a group) by a Qualified Clinical Data Registry (QCDR), Qualified Registry, or EHR/Health IT Vendor

Individual/Solo Practitioners, including
• MIPS APM participants
• Non-QP Advanced APM participants
(1 clinician billing under the TIN/SSN)
	1. Individual practitioners (or their representatives) that will be **submitting MIPS data directly** to qpp.cms.gov including data for any, or all, of the following MIPS performance categories (individual or group reporting):
	  • Quality (via file upload)
	  • Advancing Care Information (via file upload or attestation)
	  • Improvement Activities (via file upload or attestation)
	2. Individual practitioners (or their representatives) that have **secured an EHR/Health IT Vendor to submit data on their behalf** (those that are not a CMS-approved Qualified Clinical Data Registry or Qualified Registry)
	3. Individual practitioners (or their representatives) that want to **view data submitted on their behalf** by a Qualified Clinical Data Registry (QCDR), Qualified Registry, or EHR/Health IT Vendor

QCDRs **Registries** **EHR/Health IT vendors**	Third party organizations submitting MIPS data directly to qpp.cms.gov on behalf of their clients (group and/or individual clinicians) including data for any, or all of the following performance categories: • **Quality** (via QPP JSON/XML or QRDA III XML file upload) • **Advancing Care Information** (via QPP JSON/XML or QRDA III XML file upload) • **Improvement Activities** (via QPP JSON/XML or QRDA III XML file upload) **NOTE**: An EIDM role is not necessary for data submission via Application Program Interface (API) by QCDRs and Qualified Registries.

    Access Numbers (PTANs) (do not use the Group NPI or Group PTAN)

— Organization Address, City, State, Zip Code, and Phone Number

• Users requesting the **Individual Practitioner** role must provide all of the following:

— Clinician's Name

— Clinician's Medicare billing TIN

— Legal Business Name

— Clinician's Rendering NPI corresponding PTAN

— Address, City, State, Zip Code, and Phone Number

TABLE 4-4. EIDM Roles and Functions

Reporting Option	EIDM Role	EIDM Role Type	Functions
Groups, including: • MIPS APM participants • Non-QP Advanced APM participants (2+ clinicians billing under the TIN)	Security Official	Provider Approver	• Approve "PQRS Submitter" or "Web Interface Submitter" role requests by EIDM account holders for their organization (including EHR/Health IT vendors reporting on behalf of their TIN. • Submit any MIPS data on behalf of the group, either reporting as a group or for eligible clinicians reporting individually. • View all data (including PII) submitted by/on behalf of a group reporting as a group (TIN level). • View all data submitted by/on behalf of the clinicians in the practice reporting individually.
	PQRS Submitter	PQRS Provider	• Submit any non-CMS Web Interface MIPS data on behalf of the practice, either as a group or for eligible clinicians reporting individually. • View all data submitted by/on behalf of the group. • View all data submitted by/on behalf of the clinicians in the practice reporting individually. Note: An organization must have a Security Official before a user can request the PQRS Submitter role.
	Web Interface Submitter	PQRS Provider	• Submit CMS Web Interface MIPS data on behalf of the practice. • View all data submitted by/on behalf of the practice. • View all data submitted by/on behalf of the clinicians in the practice reporting individually. Note: An organization must have a Security Official before a user can request the Web Interface Submitter Role.
Individual/Solo Practitioners, including • MIPS APM participants • Non-QP Advanced APM participants (1 clinician billing under the TIN/SSN)	Individual Practitioner	Provider Approver	• Approve "PQRS Submitter" role requests by EIDM account holders for the clinician (including EHR/Health IT vendors reporting on behalf of the clinician). • Submit data on behalf of the clinician. • View all data submitted by/on behalf of the clinician.
	Individual Practitioner Representative	PQRS Provider	• Submit any MIPS data on behalf of the clinician. • View all data submitted by/on behalf of the clinician. Note: There must be a user with the Individual Practitioner role before a user can request the Individual Practitioner Representative role.

- Users requesting the **PQRS Submitter, Web Interface Submitter, or Individual Practitioner Representative** role must provide all of the following:
  — Group's Medicare billing TIN
  — Legal Business Name
  — Address, City, State, Zip Code, and Phone Number

The screenshots below are from the attestation portal built for submitting MIPS data for the 2017 performance year. The portal is expected to be updated annually to meet the reporting requirements of each performance year.

Figures 4-2A through 4-2D show the Account Dashboard for a test account. On this screen, you can see the number of APM Entities and Practices this test user is connected to. She is connected to three practices, and has the option to report on behalf of the clinicians in each practice either as a group, or as individuals.

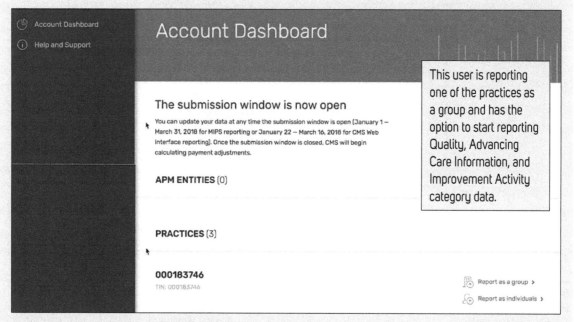

FIGURE 4-2A. QPP Attestation Account Dashboard

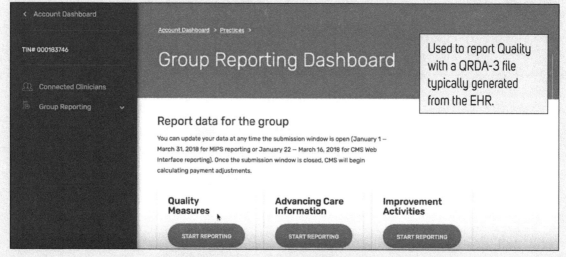

FIGURE 4-2B. QPP Attestation Account Dashboard

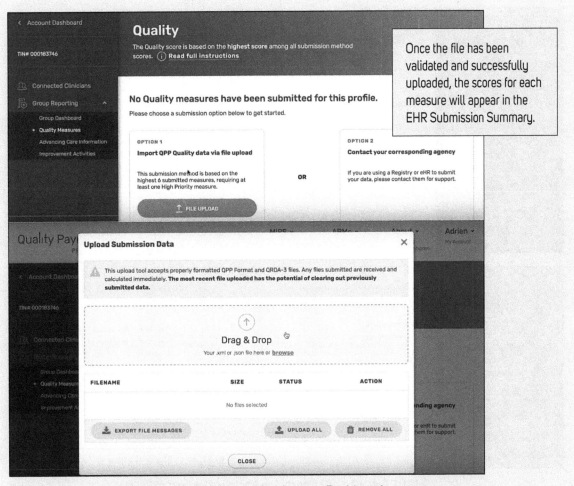

FIGURE 4-2C. QPP Attestation Account Dashboard

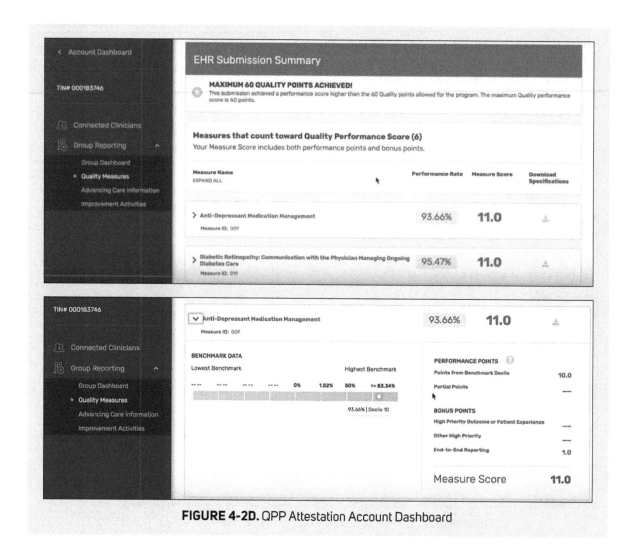

FIGURE 4-2D. QPP Attestation Account Dashboard

QUALITY—A LITTLE MORE ABOUT QRDA-3 SUBMISSIONS

There is a very specific type of file that your EHR should be able to generate that can be uploaded to the QPP attestation website to submit at least one of these three MIPS performance categories: Quality, Advancing Care Information, or Improvement Activities. These files are called Quality Reporting Data Architecture (QRDA) Type III, or QRDA-3 for short (Figure 4-3A).

The files themselves are meant to be readable more so by computers than by humans. If you happen to open one and find yourself completely bewildered by what you see, that's why. As an example, Figure 4-3B shows what the code for the "ACI Numerator Denominator Type Measure Numerator Data" looks like:

```
<observation classCode="OBS" moodCode="EVN">
    <templateId root="2.16.840.1.113883.10.20.27.3.31"
extension="2016-09-01"/>
    <code code="ASSERTION" codeSystem="2.16.840.1.113883.5.4"
codeSystemName="ActCode" displayName="Assertion"/>
    <statusCode code="completed"/>
    <value xsi:type="CD" code="NUM"
codeSystem="2.16.840.1.113883.5.4"
codeSystemName="ActCode"/>
    <!-- Numerator Count-->
    <entryRelationship typeCode="SUBJ" inversionInd="true">
        <observation classCode="OBS" moodCode="EVN">
            <templateId root="2.16.840.1.113883.10.20.27.3.3"/>
            <code code="MSRAGG" codeSystem="2.16.840.1.113883.5.4"
codeSystemName="ActCode" displayName="rate aggregation"/>
            <statusCode code="completed"/>
            <value xsi:type="INT" value="600"/>
            <methodCode code="COUNT"
codeSystem="2.16.840.1.113883.5.84"
codeSystemName="ObservationMethod" displayName="Count"/>
        </observation>
    </entryRelationship>
</observation>
```

FIGURE 4-3B. QRDA-3 File Example

For 2018, the performance period requirements include a full year of data for the Quality category, and 90 days of data for the Improvement Activities and for the Advancing Care Information performance categories. For the MIPS-eligible clinician participating as an individual, your eCQM populations include all patients (all-payer data) seen by the MIPS-eligible clinician during the performance period. For group participation, eCQM populations include all patients (all-payer data). Data submission for both individual MIPS-eligible clinicians and groups will occur between January 2, 2019 and March 31, 2019.

For all MIPS-eligible clinicians program reporting, certain identifiers are *mandatory*, meaning that they must be present in the QRDA-3 report and no nulls are allowed. Exceptions and considerations are noted where applicable. Mandatory identifiers for MIPS-eligible clinicians include:
- National Provider Identifier (NPI)
  — Required for MIPS individual reporting
  — Not allowed for MIPS group reporting
- Tax Identification Number (TIN)
  — Required for MIPS group reporting and MIPS individual reporting

Submitting data for the Advancing Care Information category has more to it. Start by selecting your performance period, choose the ACI measure set you will be reporting, find your EHR, and agree to the three attestation statements. Enter the numerator and denominator or yes/no statement for each Base, Performance, and Bonus objectives. The ACI score will update in real time at the top of the screen as you enter your data (Figures 4-4A–4-4C).

Attesting for the Improvement Activity category is similar. Select your performance period and search for your activities. For best results, search by activity ID. Once found, simply mark each activity "yes."

Advancing Care Information

Review the advancing care information measures available. Remember, in order to get credit for advancing care information, you must submit information for the required measures. (i) **Read full instructions**

⬆ FILE UPLOAD

Attestation	EHR

Start by selecting your performance period: MM/DD/YYYY 📅 To MM/DD/YYYY 📅 ❓

CHOOSING THE CORRECT ADVANCING CARE INFORMATION MEASURE SET ∧ HIDE

In 2017, there are two measure set options for reportings:
1. 2017 Advancing Care Information Transition Measures
2. Advancing Care Information Measures

Need help identifying your electronic health record technology version?

🔍 ChARM EHR ⊗ **SEARCH**

EDITION YEAR: 2014

Based on the results of your search, the edition of your product will allow you to submit measures from:

• **2017 Advancing Care Information Transition Measure Set**

When choosing the combination of technologies path, you may not submit a measure from the ACI measure set that correlates to a 2017 ACI transition measure. For example, if you submit the Provide Patient Access 2017 ACI transition measure (worth up to 20%), you may not submit the correlating ACI measures Provide Patient Access (worth up to 10%) or Patient-Generated Health Data (worth up to 10%).

NOTE: The 2015 Edition has the reporting capability to support either the 2017 Advancing Care Information Transition Measures or the Advancing Care Information Measures. We encourage clinicians and vendors that collect and combine data from the 2014 and 2015 Editions during a performance period to aggregate their numerators and denominators for the 2017 Advancing Care Information Transition Measures.

Select Measure Set:

2017 ADVANCING CARE INFORMATION TRANSITION MEASURES	ADVANCING CARE INFORMATION MEASURES	COMBINATION OF BOTH MEASURE SETS

ATTESTATION STATEMENTS FOR THE ADVANCING CARE INFORMATION PERFORMANCE CATEGORY ❓

> **Prevention of Information Blocking Attestation**	Yes	No
> **ONC Direct Review Attestation**	Yes	No
> **ONC-ACB Surveillance Attestation (Optional)**	Yes	No

FIGURE 4-4A.

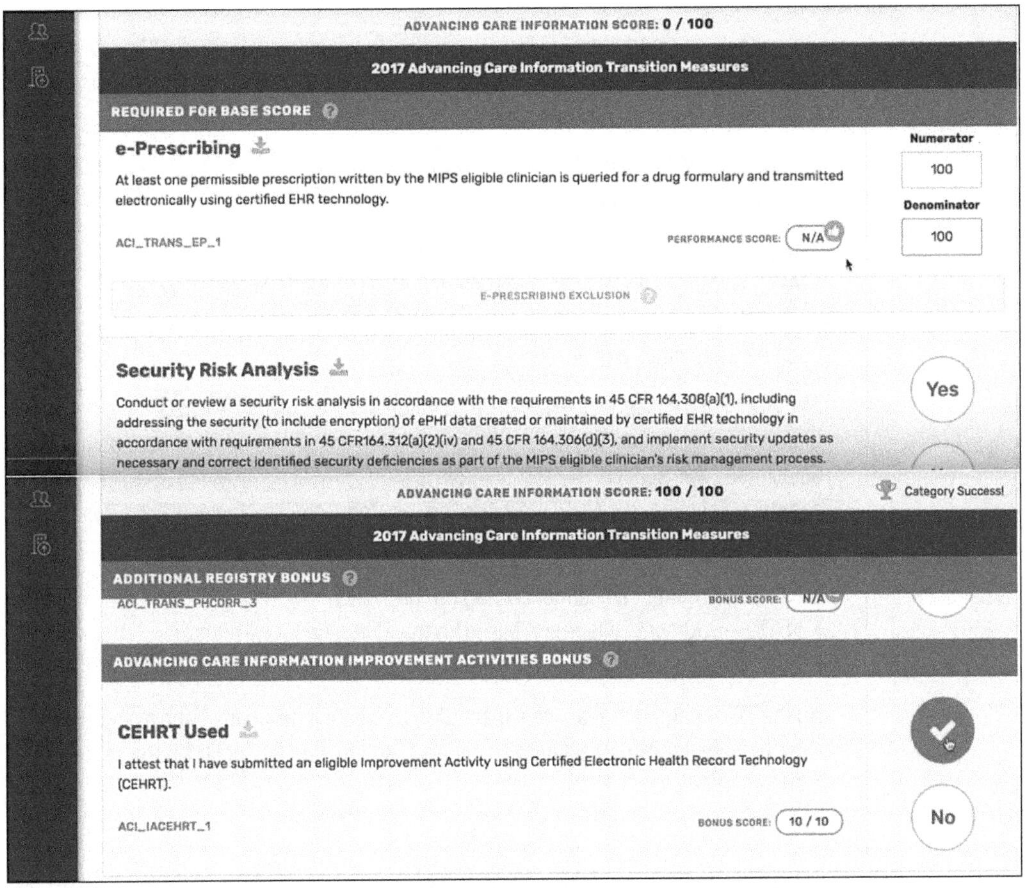

FIGURE 4-4B.

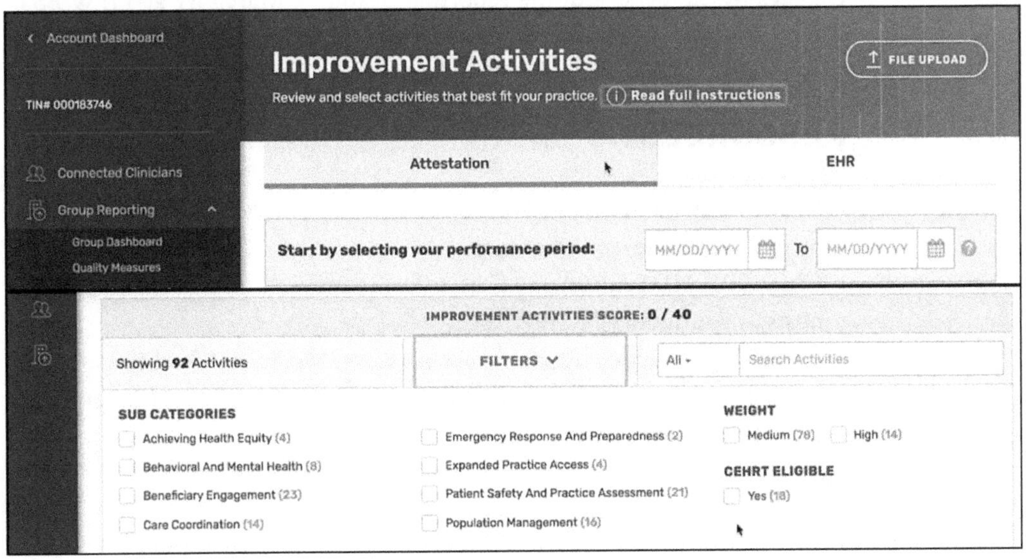

FIGURE 4-4C.

Once it's all said and done, your data is submitted, feedback given, time has passed, and it's time to receive your payment adjustment. Here's the big question: what will it look like?

In the past, CMS would add a code to your remittance advice to inform you which program was associated with the reduction in payment.

A claim adjustment reason code (CARC) and a remittance advice remark code (RARC) are code sets used to report payment adjustments on an individual clinician's or group practice's Remittance Advice. Both of these code sets are updated three times a year.

The PQRS, EHR Incentive Program, and Value Modifier used CARC 237—Legislated/Regulatory Penalty to designate when a negative or downward payment adjustment was applied. At least one Remark Code must be provided (may be comprised of either the NCPDP Reject Reason Code, or Remittance Advice Remark Code that is not an ALERT) in combination with the following RARCs:

- N699—Payment adjustment based on the PQRS
- N700—Payment adjustment based on the EHR Incentive Program
- N701—Payment adjustment based on the Value-based Payment Modifier

By the 2019 payment year, we expect CMS to create a new code to be associated with the negative MIPS payment adjustment, and for it to be applied in the same manner.

Note, there is no official submission button. Information is automatically saved. The attestation portal remains open and allows for unlimited changes to the data until the reporting deadline, March 31 at 11:59 EST, when the numbers and statements in the system are considered final.

RESOURCES

- Group and/or Individual data submission for MIPS training video: https://youtu.be/q0Cvke6fnrg
- CMS QPP APM Advancing Care Information Submission training video: https://youtu.be/yTR5l9yCmOI
- EIDM User Guide: https://www.cms.gov/Medicare/Quality-Payment-Program/Resource-Library/Enterprise-Identity-Data-Management-EIDM-User-Guide.pdf

CHAPTER 5

Public Reporting

We've discussed in detail how MIPS is a comparative and competitive program. However, the MIPS Score is worth much more than just penalty avoidance and earning exceptional performance bonus. It will soon represent every eligible clinician's pubic report card, since CMS mandated that MIPS scores of all eligible clinicians would be made public on the Physician Compare website, located at www.medicare.gov/physiciancompare.

Physician Compare encourages consumers to make informed choices while also incentivizing physicians to maximize their performance. The site already offers consumers the ability to browse through Medicare healthcare providers nationwide, by searching:

- Basic demographic info
- Medical School education and residency info
- Primary and secondary specialty
- Board certification (if any)
- Practice and hospital affiliations
- Languages spoken
- Whether the provider attested to MU, participated in PQRS, and committed to the Million Hearts initiative in the most recent year
- For group practices, a complete list of other physicians in the group, by specialty
- Geography
- Health problem

CMS will soon be adding the following MIPS information on Physician Compare: Complete Performance Scores, performance category scores, and aggregate information on MIPS, which includes the range of final scores for all MIPS-eligible clinicians and the range of performance of all the MIPS-eligible clinicians for each performance category.

CMS will add these data each year to Physician Compare for each MIPS-eligible clinician or group, either on the profile pages or in the downloadable database.

At the time of this writing, only performance data from the PQRS program was publicly available on the site. However, it will only become more robust over time. To give you an idea of the current state of the site, the following page features a de-identified screenshot for both an individual and a group profile (Figure 5-1).

Data from the 2017 program year is expected to be available for public reporting in late 2018, while data from the 2018 program year is expected to be available for public reporting in late 2019. This will include:

- All measures under the Quality performance category
- A subset of cost measures that meet the public reporting standards
- All activities under the MIPS improvement activities performance category
- An indicator on Physician Compare for any eligible clinician or group who successfully meets the ACI performance category

Any ACI objectives, activities, or measures must meet the public reporting standards applicable to data posted on Physician Compare.

CMS uses the Achievable Benchmark of Care (ABC™) methodology to determine a benchmark for the quality, cost, improvement activities, and ACI data. This benchmark is then used as the basis of a five-star rating for each available measure. The ABCTM benchmark helps patients and caregivers interpret the data accurately and has been historically well received by the clinicians and entities it measures.

It's important to distinguish that only those measures that meet the public reporting standards will be considered for benchmarking and star ratings, and the benchmark will be based on the most recently available data each year.

Also, clinicians and groups who voluntarily opt-in to MIPS, even when they can be excluded will be offered a 30-day preview period, and have the option to opt out of having their data publicly reported on Physician Compare.

Since the website's launch in 2010, CMS has been continually working to:

- Enhance the site and its functionality
- Improve the information available
- Include more and increasingly useful information about physicians and other health care professionals who participate in Medicare

The criteria for being listed on Physician Compare is outlined below in Table 5-1.

Keep in mind, the data available on Physician Compare can be procured for free by third party physician rating websites, such as Health Grades,

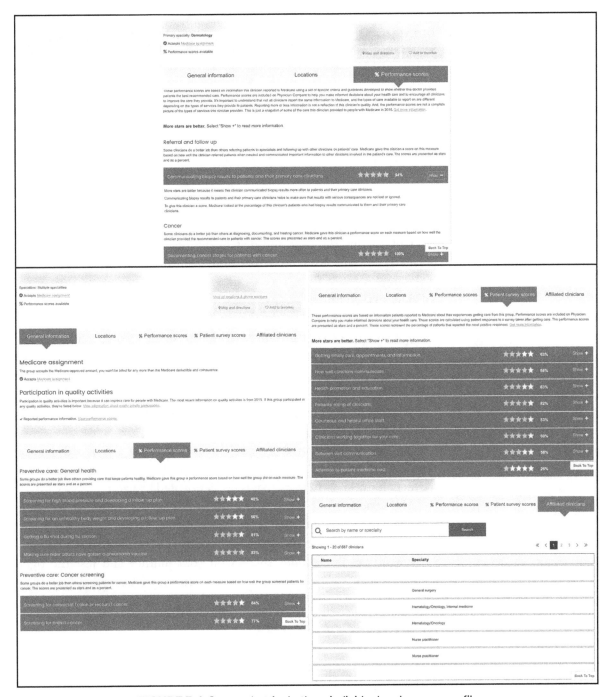

FIGURE 5-1. Screenshot for both an individual and a group profile

Yelp, and Google. So even if your patients are not aware of the Physician Compare website, the data presented there will be made available throughout the internet.

TABLE 5-1. Physician Compare Criteria

Health care professionals must:	Group practices must:
Be in approved status in PECOS	Be in approved status in PECOS
Provide at least one practice location address	Have a legal business name
Have at least one specialty noted in PECOS	Have a valid practice location address
Have submitted a Medicare fee-for-service claim within the last 12 months or be newly enrolled in PECOS within the last 6 months	Have at least two active Medicare health professionals reassign their benefits to the group's TIN
	Have submitted a Medicare fee-for-service claim within the last 12 months or be newly enrolled in PECOS within the last 6 months

Considering the near and distant futures, a high MIPS score could present clinicians with more bargaining power in multiple situations, including:

- Clinician recruitment
- Mergers, acquisitions, and sale of practices
- Negotiating fees with private healthcare insurance companies who are using value-based contracts

****

"I am in favor of progress; it's change I don't like."
– Mark Twain

No one said any of this would be easy. Among the already hectic demands of being a clinician, preparing for the shift to a merit-based payment model is hard work that is detail oriented by nature.

My Advice:

Learn the rules of the game, so you know where you can strategically focus or relax your efforts without compromising your score or reputation.

I wish you tremendous success on your journey and just the right amount of luck!

GLOSSARY OF TERMS

ABC—Achievable Benchmark of Care
ACI—Advancing Care Information
ACO—Accountable Care Organization
API—Application Programming Interface
APM—Alternate Payment Model
BMI—Body Mass Index
CAHPS—Consumer Assessment of Health Plans Study

CARC—Claim Adjustment Reason Code
C-CDA—Consolidated Clinical Data Architecture
CEHRT—Certified EHR Technology
CMS—Centers for Medicare and Medicaid
CQM—Clinical Quality Measure
EC—Eligible Clinician
eCQM—electronic-Clinical Quality Measure
EHR—Electronic Health Record
EIDM—Enterprise Identity Data Management
HHS—Health and Human Services
HIE—Health Information Exchange
ICD—Internal Classification of Diseases
IA—Improvement Activities
MAC—Medicare Administrative Contractor
MACRA—Medicare Authorization and CHIP Reimbursement Act
MIPS—Merit-based Incentive Payment System
MSPB—Medicare Spending Per Beneficiary
NPI—National Provider Identifier
PECOS—Provider Electronic Chain Online System
PCP—Primary Care Physician
PGHD—Patient-generated Health Data
PQRS—Physician Quality Reporting System
QCDR—Qualified Clinical Data Registry
QDC—Quality Data Code
QP—Qualifying Participant (APMs)
QPP—Quality Payment Program
QRDA—Quality Reporting Document Architecture
QRUR—Quality and Resource Use Report
PTAN—Provider Transaction Access Numbers
RAF—Risk Adjustment Factor
RARC—Remittance Advice Remark Code
SGR—Sustainable Growth Rate
SSN—Social Security Number
TIN—Tax Identification Number
VDT—View, Download, Transmit
VM—Value-based Modifier

CPSIA information can be obtained
at www.ICGtesting.com
Printed in the USA
BVHW06s1434220418
513925BV00001B/1/P

9 780999 355381